DANGEROUS MEDICINE

9/10/13

Daniel,

   Please enjoy, but you must read it!

[signature]

P.S. Too bad we couldn't continue
our show "Health Secrets"

DANGEROUS MEDICINE

WHAT YOUR DOCTOR DOESN'T KNOW CAN HURT YOU

Ken G. Knott, M.D.

Youth Enhancement Systems, Inc.

Dangerous Medicine

ISBN: 978-0-9855105-0-

Library of Congress Control Number: 2012937695

TABLE OF CONTENTS

FOREWORD

Dr. Ken Knott has written a very important book. He is a Board-Certified orthopedic medicine physician who became fed up with many of conventional medicine's practices. Instead of giving in to his frustrations, Dr. Knott took a different path: he searched for safe and effective natural therapies that work in a clinical practice. This book is a compilation of his research and practice.

Hypothyroidism is occurring at epidemic rates. Over forty percent of people may have an undiagnosed, abnormal thyroid condition. The consequences of hypothyroidism are severe: heart attacks, excessive fatigue, strokes, and mental decline. Dr. Knott clearly shows the failure in conventional medicine's reliance on laboratory testing as the sole means to diagnose a hypothyroid condition.

Hypothyroidism can affect every cell in the body. The thyroid hormone exerts its influence inside each and every one of the trillions of cells in the human body. Conventional blood tests do not measure the function of thyroid hormone inside the cells. Why should we be relying on a test that does not measure the true function of thyroid hormone? Dr. Knott makes a strong point that the diagnosis of hypothyroidism is a clinical diagnosis best made with a combination of obtaining a good history and physical examination along with having patients measure their basal body temperatures. Finally, correlating that data with appropriate thyroid blood tests provides a more accurate picture of thyroid status as compared to relying solely on blood tests.

Dr. Knott reviews all the endocrine glands and why natural, bioidentical hormones can be an effective regimen for helping a patient overcome chronic illness as well as achieving his/her optimal health. He reviews conditions like andropause and menopause and how to safely and effectively treat the symptoms from these conditions.

I see adrenal fatigue occurring in a large percentage of my patients. These are the patients suffering from fatigue, headaches, and brain fog. Dr. Knott reviews the adrenal hormones and how natural versions of these hormones can dramatically improve one's health.

Much more than hormones are contained in this book. Dr. Knott shows which micronutrients are effective and why we have become so deficient in various vitamins and minerals. He describes the effectiveness of other therapies such as hyperbaric oxygen and prolotherapy. Conventional medicine offers drugs and surgery for most of our health problems. Dr. Knott offers a different approach. This approach is at odds with Big Pharma. Dr. Knott shows you why Big Pharma is against these safe and effective approaches.

I highly recommend this book for all people, especially those over the age of forty, who are searching for safe and effective natural therapies that work. Dr. Knott has a lifetime of experience that he shares with all of us. This book should be read by doctors and patients alike.

-David Brownstein, M.D.

Author of eleven books including: *Iodine: Why You Need It, Why You Can't Live Without It, The Miracle of Natural Hormones,* and *Overcoming Thyroid Disorders.* Dr. Brownstein also authors his monthly newsletter, *Dr. Brownstein's Natural Way to Health.* More information can be found at www.drbrownstein.com.

PREFACE

A number of my friends, other doctors, and patients urged me to share my thoughts about what I have learned and know about optimizing health. The key phrase to remember is *what I have learned and know about optimizing health* because I am not making any claim that I know everything. To the contrary, there are many things about achieving optimum health that remain speculative at best or unknown. This book considers many of the things that I have been found to be supported by science and practical application, regardless of popular opinion or so-called standards of practice. Accordingly, after many months of coaxing, I decided to reduce to writing the things I have been teaching other doctors and telling my patients for years. Many will ask, "Why doesn't my doctor know that?" The answer to that question will vary, but it typically involves the central theme of not being properly educated on many of the subjects covered. Some of you will not accept that answer as being correct because it is understandable that everyone wants to believe that their doctor knows everything and would never stretch the truth in order to save face. To understand my answer more completely, you first have to understand the training system for doctors in this country.

In order to become a doctor, one must not only obtain a college degree, but that process must take place with honors and grade-point averages (GPAs) that are superior to the majority of students. Medical colleges typically exclude any applicant if their GPAs are not in the superior range. One of the other requirements for consideration is to take the Medical College Admission Test (MCAT). Again, if that score is not in the top 10th percentile range, a student will usually not be considered for admission to a medical college. Even if a student makes excellent grades and scores highly on the MCAT exam, that still doesn't guarantee enrollment in a medical college. Additional factors are considered, including student involvement in extracurricular activities such as honor societies or scholastic clubs. Did the applicant hold an office in any of those organizations? Did he or she work while attending school? Does he or she have letters of recommendation from doctors or other leaders of the medical community? If a student makes the grade, then he/she is in the position of competing with hundreds of other similar students, all of whom want to go to medical school. If the student applicant makes it that far, then they must meet admissions committee members personally for interviews. Only a small percentage of medical school applicants are accepted and offered a place in a medical college class, so one can begin to see the odds that must be overcome just to make it that far.

When a student has been accepted and begins his/her medical education, that's when the real work begins, as they are bombarded with an overload of information. They are expected to remember everything about every subject having to do with the human body and the many things that cause health problems including injuries and diseases. By the time a medical student has successfully completed his/her first year of medical school, he/she has accomplished something educationally that most people never have the opportunity or willingness to achieve. As a result, many medical students begin to develop an attitude that they know more than most people, and some develop varying degrees of superiority or downright arrogance. Furthermore, once a student has been accepted into a medical school, he/she justifiably believes most of what is being taught is correct, since they are involved with what they have been conditioned to believe is the epitome of the educational process. Consider this: **some of what medical students are taught is wrong,** regardless of whether or not they think they have arrived at the epitome of education!

One of the basic science courses taught is pharmacology which is a study of prescription medications, including their indications, actions, dosage, and side effects. The only courses given about nutrition are limited and barely touch the surface. Accordingly, there is little wonder that most physicians accept what they are told in regard to nutrition and scoff at the mention of home remedies that have a connection. That lack of information and training has led to the continuing myth, among many others, that cholesterol causes heart disease. There are still doctors who recommend low fat diets for heart patients and continue to prescribe statin drugs to reduce cholesterol levels. Statin drugs are dangerous, but millions of Americans have been convinced by their doctors to take this class of drugs. If anyone has concerns about whether or not to take a statin drug, I suggest they read the product insert section about side effects.

Once students successfully complete four years of medical school, they then graduate with an M.D. (Medical Doctor) or D.O. (Doctor of Osteopathy) degree. There is virtually no difference between the two degrees other than the title because the training is essentially identical.

The graduate doctor then, in the majority of cases, begins specialty training in a chosen field and that further compounds the problem of misinformation when a doctor is trained incorrectly. Specialty training is superior in many ways, but incorrect or obsolete information continues to be taught and is accepted as fact. Most specialist doctors proceed with blind obedience to what they learned and simply refuse to apply logic when necessary. Once these doctors have completed four years of medical college and four or more years of specialty training, most will typically close their minds to anything that is considered foreign or in disagreement with what they have already learned. That is a dangerous combination, but it is a fact of life with most doctors. A true scientist remains open-minded and doctors are supposed to be scientists. Unfortunately, for the reasons given, many doctors are very close-minded and are very reluctant to change their way of thinking, regardless of the rationale. That is unacceptable at best and deadly at worst. Doctors are people, and most people are resistant to change. Change often means work or additional thought. After years of training, why should they change their way of thinking, particularly when they earnestly believe everything they learned was correct?

Another problem with doctors is for them to admit they are wrong. It may not be a virtue, but that's the way it is in many cases. Throughout their educational career, all doctors are rewarded to be right, not wrong! Instead of admitting a mistake or a lack of information, many physicians ridicule or speak against alternative methods or subjects that lie outside their fund of knowledge. As a result, the situation can arise that can put your health and life in jeopardy, because it's what your doctor doesn't know that can hurt you.

The very specialty that should be providing direction for metabolic disorders, endocrinology, is the same specialty that has failed to take the lead and impeded progress, in many cases, by adhering to sometimes antiquated and useless tests and treatment methods. If a new paradigm does not fit within the fund of knowledge and thinking of most endocrinologists, then it must be wrong in their opinion. That is very unfortunate, because some of the finest and most astute physicians that I have had the pleasure of knowing were trained in endocrinology. There are many doctors in positions of authority who personify the definition of being close-minded, and it is the patients that ultimately suffer as a result. I refer to these types of doctors, regardless of their chosen specialty, as members of the "Flat Earth Society."

Historical evidence has shown that most people began to believe that the earth was round as far back as the time of

Ptolemy and Aristotle. For the most part, the only group that continued to promote the idea that the earth was the center of the universe was the Catholic Church. By the mid-1600s, it had been established that the earth was not flat and rotated around the sun. The Catholic Church forced scientists to denounce their beliefs as heresy. It is this blind adherence to antiquated and unproven ideas that is so dangerous. Any physician who adheres to antiquated and disputed ideas, in spite of overwhelming evidence to the contrary, automatically becomes a member of the "Flat Earth Society." If you don't think there are such doctors, all you have to do is watch some of them on nationally syndicated talk shows when they speak poorly about what is currently referred to as **anti-aging medicine.**

Anti-aging medicine is more of a philosophy than a specialty. Other than the recent attempts to extend the life of telomeres, there is nothing currently available that will reverse or delay the aging process. So the term "anti-aging medicine" may be somewhat of a misnomer. I prefer a more appropriate term, "age management," which simply implies that the emphasis will be upon managing the variable factors that may optimize a person's health as they age. The major factor, regarding how fast one ages, is genetically determined. At this time, there is no method by which one can change the genetic code that allows for a longer life, and one must accept the cards they were dealt. My focus is to improve my patients' quality of life with proper hormonal balance, nutrition, and exercise. It stands to reason that a healthier person will live longer, but the jury is still out since the field remains in its infancy.

I have often been asked the question as to why I am so knowledgeable about nutrition and hormonal replacement being that my board certification is in Physical Medicine and Rehabilitation (PM&R) instead of endocrinology. That's actually a very good question, as most specialists in my field have no more knowledge about nutrition or hormonal replacement than most other doctors. For those of you who don't recognize the specialty of PM&R, I will explain. After medical school, I completed a rotating surgical internship and then completed an additional multi-year training program in PM&R at The Ohio State University. After successfully completing the training program, I underwent the appropriate written and oral examinations and became board certified. Once a doctor becomes board certified, that is as far as he/she can go in that particular field of medicine unless they choose to sub-specialize in one of the aspects of their field. PM&R is actually two specialties in one. The first is Physical Medicine and the name was given because of the many "physical" agents that we use to treat injuries or disease. Examples of physical agents are injections, such as an epidural, and other physical agents including ice, heat in various forms, exercise, range of motion, balance/gait training, conservation techniques, traction, etc. PM&R is the only specialty that teaches, as an integral part of the specialty training program, various physical modalities that are typically referred to as physical therapy. Years ago, these physical medicine modalities were taught to assistants since the doctors had far too busy schedules to perform those treatments personally. As a result, the field of physical therapy was born. The other half of the specialty is Rehabilitation Medicine. It is concerned primarily with the treatment of patients with spinal cord injuries, head injuries, strokes, multiple sclerosis, muscular dystrophy, cerebral palsy, collagen vascular diseases such as rheumatoid arthritis, lupus, and other diseases or conditions of the central or peripheral nervous system. Rehabilitation doctors spend much of their time in hospitals because many of their patients have been severely injured or are seriously ill requiring hospitalization and intensive care. I chose the path of Physical Medicine, but have been fully trained in all aspects of my specialty.

So how and why did I learn and evolve my practice to include hormone replacement therapy and nutrition? There were a variety of factors that pushed me in that direction, but the main reason was something that simply happened by chance. In 1993, a forty-eight-year-old lady was referred to me by an orthopedic surgeon after having seen eight other physicians. She had twisted her knee over two years before and no one could determine why her knee continued to remain swollen and excruciatingly painful. She could not tolerate bearing weight and came to me with the intent of undergoing prolotherapy (to be explained later). My instinct told me that she was one of the patients who would not respond to prolotherapy, but at the time, I didn't know why. I just knew that some patients didn't respond as well as others. Nothing could be found to explain why her problem had not resolved, but for all intents and purposes, her life as a productive useful person was over. I knew something was missing and I just couldn't put my finger on it; but as luck would have it, I decided not to inject her knee. Shortly thereafter, I attended a medical conference in a western U.S. city where a physician friend of mine resided. I contacted him while I was there. I asked him about my forty-eight-year-old female patient with unexplained knee pain and swelling. He asked if she was post menopausal and I told him that she had undergone a total hysterectomy some five years prior to seeing me. Without deep thought or hesitation, he asked about her level of testosterone. I told him that I didn't think anyone had tested it and he acted very surprised. At the time, I didn't understand his reaction so I asked him why he wanted to know about her testosterone level and he replied with a question, "Don't any of you know that it's the major hormone for healing?" I knew about the anabolic capacity of testosterone, but I never put it together and certainly not in a female. When I returned to Atlanta, I called the patient and made arrangements for her to be tested. I didn't place much credence with what my older friend had told me, so I dismissed it from my mind thinking to myself that I had managed to humor him by getting the test done. When the test result came back, it read, "NONE DETECTED." Because of what I had not learned in medical school or residency training, I tried to convince myself that the test results were a fluke and meant very little, but I was still somewhat surprised. I called my friend who immediately said, "NONE DETECTED, right?" It was at that time that I truly began to believe that he might actually be onto something that everyone had missed, but I still didn't want to admit that ten reputable doctors had all missed this. I said to him, "How did you know that?" and he said, "Ken, if you're still practicing medicine when you are seventy-three years of age like me, you should know a few more things about medicine than your younger colleagues and this is just one of those things. Just be glad you didn't inject her knee because it wouldn't have healed." Needless to say, I was dumbfounded, but aware that I had just learned something important. He advised me that no one knows it all, but told me to learn from what he had just taught me. He asked what I thought I should do in a woman without any measurable level of testosterone. I decided to research the issue myself and was somewhat surprised to find that not a lot had been written on the subject, but I read enough to make an educated guess. I was very concerned because I had never prescribed testosterone for a female patient before. She called my office about 5-6 weeks later crying hysterically. She refused to leave a message and insisted on talking to me. I began to think the worst, but I answered the call. Once she regained some composure, she began telling me a story that she did not tell me when we first met. She and her husband were formerly involved in ballroom dancing, were widely known in those circles, and had won several championships nationwide. She continued with her story by telling me that she had not been able to walk, much less dance, since she had injured her knee. She then said, "I went dancing for the first time in over two years last Saturday night. My knee pain is gone and I wanted to thank you for what you have done for me." I was totally surprised, but I had enough composure to say, "I'm so glad you're better." My mind was spinning because so many things were going through it at that point, such as why I had never learned that in my training. I was shocked, surprised, ashamed, and angry that everyone, including me, had missed that simple hormonal deficiency. My older doctor friend was right, I had learned something that opened new doors for me and changed my professional life.

Since that time, I have dedicated myself to learning as much about this fascinating subject as possible. Since 2006, I have been teaching other doctors about hormonal replacement and nutrition and spend as much time as possible learning more by reading, attending courses, and associating with others who are true experts. I have met a number of truly great doctors and scientists to whom I owe a great deal. Dr. Barry Sears and Drs. Mike and Mary Dan Eades were instrumental in teaching me more about nutrition than I would have ever learned otherwise. Dr. Therese Hertogue is another important person who has helped me tremendously in my quest for knowledge along with Drs. David Brownstein and Diana Schwarzbein. I have been able to keep an open mind and that has enabled my learning process. The mind truly is like a parachute, neither works unless they are open.

Don't be a victim of a "Flat Earth Society" doctor because it is truly still your choice. Remember that these types are located throughout the field of medicine in all specialties, and can occupy positions of influence and prominence within learning institutions. It could also be your own family doctor! Beware of that type regardless of who they are or what their chosen specialty is, because it is what they don't know or are unwilling to learn that can hurt you.

How would you know that your own doctor is up-to-speed on the subject of age management medicine? There are a number of ways to determine that and many will be covered in succeeding chapters, but if your doctor is unwilling to listen or ridicules you for touching on the subject, then you should run, not walk, from his/her office. Also, if they repeat some of the myths associated with hormone replacement or nutrition, it's a sure bet they won't be open to the type of discussion you want. I plan to provide a nationwide list of doctors on my web site **www.managingyourage.com**. This list is incomplete, but it's a start.

As I indicated, there are many ways to seek out a doctor who is up to date, knowledgeable, and open-minded about age management medicine. The following examples will provide a few clues. Endocrinology is a wonderful and interesting specialty, but for the most part, doctors in that specialty have missed the boat in regards to age management. There are a few very knowledgeable endocrinologists who are among some of the finest age management physicians available. However, one must be very careful when selecting a doctor, regardless of his/her credentials. If a doctor refuses to talk to you about natural bio-identical hormonal replacement, my advice would be to not return to that office. There is a difference between the hormones your body has made for your entire life as compared to chemical look-alikes. Doctors who prefer to use chemicals instead of bio-identical hormones should be avoided. A doctor who tells you that you're just "getting old" is another type to avoid, as are those who say you're in the "normal range" and don't need treatment, regardless of your symptoms. Normal is quite different than optimal, but few doctors recognize that fact, as little is written about the subject. Doctors who don't recognize the thyroid as the most important endocrine organ should be avoided, as should those who base a diagnosis and treatment strictly upon the results of a lab study. Avoid doctors who ignore you and your symptoms and only are interested in your laboratory results. Choose a doctor who will treat you, not the labs! Be concerned if a doctor ridicules the anti-aging field. If you are female, understand that you need hormones after menopause, regardless of whether or not you still have your uterus and regardless of whether or not you are experiencing hot flashes and night sweats. If you are male, beware of the doctor who does not routinely check your estradiol (estrogen) or tells you that your testosterone is normal for your age.

True science dictates that we seek legitimate methods to improve quality of life and maintain health. It's in accordance with the oath taken by all doctors as well as being morally sound. So why is there so much opposition to this very simple concept? First, physicians in positions of authority have ascribed to certain concepts, regardless of their validity, and changing an opinion takes effort and a willingness to admit an error. Many of these same people have spent their professional lives securing grants and performing studies that are published in recognized medical journals. In order to secure such grants to pay for those studies, the involved doctors must continue playing the same game. In academic medicine, there is a saying, "publish or perish." To explain, it means that doctors are viewed more favorably when they publish more studies. Unfortunately, it is the quality of studies that is of most importance, not the quantity. I say unfortunately because many academic physicians place a much higher value upon quantity and, as a result, the quality suffers and can lead to intellectual dishonesty. Examples of this type of occurrence are the studies by Dr. Ancel Keys that will be discussed in the chapter, "You Are What You Eat." His studies were poorly designed and led to the decades old fallacy that dietary fat caused heart disease. Instead of retracting statements or changing a position, it is much easier to maintain the status quo and continue receiving grant money and stipends. As a result, these same "experts" must disagree with any theory differing with their own, hence the reason for the dogmatic stance on various issues, including those regarding the metabolism and diet.

The foregoing are but a few things to consider when choosing a doctor. I only mention this because the choice is of utmost importance as, I will repeat again, it's what your doctor doesn't know that can hurt you.

1

THE IMPORTANCE OF THE THYROID FOR OPTIMAL HEALTH

Traditional testing and treatment for the thyroid has gone overboard in the wrong direction. For such a tiny organ, the thyroid gland holds the esteemed position of being the most important of the endocrine glands. Located just below the thyroid cartilage (Adam's apple) and cricoid cartilage, it is butterfly in shape and wraps around the trachea (windpipe) in the front of the lower part of the neck. It also has smaller glands associated with it, specifically parathyroid glands, which secrete calcitonin; a chemical necessary for calcium metabolism and proper bony mineralization.

Dr. William Gull was the first to recognize hypothyroidism (low thyroid function) in 1874. As a result, the condition was originally referred to as "Gull's Disease." He observed a condition known as myxedema associated with a "cretinoid state" as the result of hypothyroidism.[1] Myxedema is characterized by the abnormal accumulation of a mucoid mixture of subcutaneous (under the skin) connective tissue. It gives an appearance of thickness and swelling (edema). It is also associated with dry skin, hair loss, and a reduction of mental function. The cretinoid state is derived from the syndrome, cretinism—seen in some children—and is caused by low thyroid. It is characterized by short stature and mental retardation. Dr. Gull observed many of these symptoms in those who had undergone the removal of their thyroid after childhood. In 1890, doctors transplanted the thyroid tissue from a sheep into a female patient with myxedema. The patient showed dramatic improvement of her edema, speech, movements, and energy. The method of supplementing the thyroid was improved and the first injection of thyroid extract was performed in 1891 by Dr. George Murray.[2] A year later, doctors reported giving sheep thyroid extract by mouth, which was also effective in reversing hypothyroidism.[3] [4] Oral thyroid extract was first standardized in 1895 and thyroxine, (T4) was isolated nineteen years later in 1914 by Dr. Kendall.[5] [6]The chemical structure of T4 was identified in 1926, but there was confusion about which form of T4 was more active.[7] During that time, doctors examined and observed patients and diagnosed them by interpreting complaints and physical findings. Resting body temperatures were very important in the diagnoses. It was well known and accepted that hypothyroid patients typically had suboptimal body temperatures in addition to many of the other known symptoms and signs. In 1949, thyroxine was first synthesized in a laboratory.[8] Three years later in 1952, triiodothyronine (T3) was isolated.[9] It was also determined that T3 was the dominant hormone, having a physiologic potency of four to five times that of T4.

At that time, doctors considered the many symptoms of hypothyroidism and paid close attention to the physical findings on examination in order to make a diagnosis of hypothyroidism. When most of those patients underwent replacement with desiccated thyroid preparations, their symptoms would improve. Laboratories began to develop tests to help physicians make the diagnosis, but most of those tests have proven themselves to be inadequate at best and misleading in most cases. Doctors have learned to test free T4 instead of free T3. It has been proven that it is the free portion of the T3 hormone that is primarily responsible for the body's response to thyroid. By far, the most important thyroid test is the level of free T3, but most doctors never learned that importance. Thyroid Stimulating Hormone (TSH) is considered the "gold standard" test used by most doctors, but again, it only reveals a small part of the overall picture. Even if a doctor was to obtain the most important test available (free T3), the range given by labs is grossly inaccurate because it is based upon a sample population composed of a very high percentage of patients with low thyroid function. As a result, many patients remain **untreated or under-treated** simply because of the inadequacy of the current laboratory tests. Doctors living and practicing during the time that the thyroid was being initially studied would probably scoff at the tests of today that are supposedly the gold standard. Furthermore, the doctors of that time would treat patients today whose tests are normal but are obviously hypothyroid. One would think that the treatment for hypothyroidism would have improved over the years; however, that is not the case now simply because it is traditional to rely upon commonly accepted test results while ignoring the patient's complaints and symptoms.

The thyroid gland itself secretes two important hormones, T4 and T3. T1 and T2 are also secreted, but neither have any importance other than combining to form a small percentage of T3. Reverse T3 and T4 are chemically similar, but have no positive biological activity. The "reverse" designation simply refers to the chemical configuration because the molecules are a mirror image of the active molecules. The number after the "T" designates the number of iodine atoms that are present in that molecule. T3 has three atoms of iodine attached to a thyroglobulin molecule, while T4 has four atoms of iodine. T4 is the primary hormone secreted by the thyroid as compared to T3. Most T3 results from the conversion of T4 in the liver, kidneys, and other peripheral tissues.

In a perfect world, the thyroid secretes the perfect amount of both hormones and exactly the right amount of T3 is converted from T4. The reality is that the world is not perfect and the incidence of low thyroid function (hypothyroidism) is much higher than most experts suspect. It is much more common than traditional medicine would have us believe, and actually has become an epidemic that wreaks havoc on the health of millions. In turn, this affects our whole society in terms of expensive testing, and ill-advised use of multiple drugs to treat symptoms; not to mention the associated misery for the people with hypothyroidism. It is impossible to estimate the cost associated with the condition of hypothyroidism simply because the problem has never been studied properly. If one could determine the number of missed work days alone that have resulted from the miserable circumstance of untreated or under-treated hypothyroidism, the estimated cost would be hundreds of millions, if not billions, of dollars annually. Add to that the cost of prescription drugs designed to treat the symptoms brought about as the result of hypothyroidism, and one can begin to see the tremendous importance of getting this situation under proper scientific control.

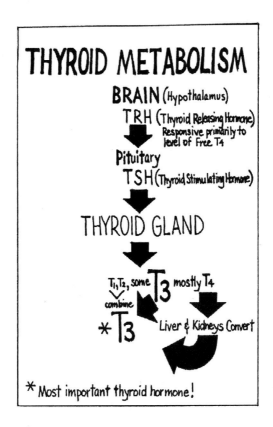

The key phrase is "scientific control." Presently, several unscientific myths continue to circulate about both hypo and hyperthyroid conditions. The first issue involves the diagnosis of either condition, but since low thyroid function or hypothyroidism is the most common condition affecting the thyroid, I will address the diagnosis of hypothyroidism.

Hypothyroidism has many symptoms, but many doctors rely upon traditional testing that is inadequate and misleading at best as noted before. Doctors must and should look at the patient and consider the symptoms that they have, but that most important basic aspect is often overlooked because of the improper way doctors have been trained to assess thyroid function. The most common symptom of low thyroid function is unexplained fatigue. Even with long periods of sleep, the hypothyroid person just never seems to have any energy. They wake up tired, stay tired throughout the day, and go to bed tired. There are certainly other causes of fatigue, but hypothyroidism is at the top of the list. Other symptoms include:

- ❖ Weight gain
- ❖ Inability to lose weight even with dietary changes
- ❖ Dry skin
- ❖ Brittle nails
- ❖ Constipation
- ❖ High blood pressure
- ❖ Eczema
- ❖ Hair loss
- ❖ Loss of outer third of eye brows
- ❖ Easy bruising
- ❖ Allergies to many things in the environment
- ❖ Feeling of being cold
- ❖ Cold hands and feet
- ❖ Mental "fog"

- ❖ Poor memory
- ❖ Difficulty concentrating
- ❖ Headaches
- ❖ Depression
- ❖ Muscle aches and pains (fibromyalgia)
- ❖ Joint aches and pains (arthritis)
- ❖ Difficulty swallowing
- ❖ Swelling of the tongue
- ❖ Impaired healing
- ❖ Frequent colds or flu-like symptoms
- ❖ Weak heart beat
- ❖ Slow pulse
- ❖ Accumulation of subcutaneous (under the skin) mucoid tissue (myxedema.)
- ❖ Cellulite
- ❖ Infertility
- ❖ Heavy menstrual flow
- ❖ Painful menstrual periods

I have treated many patients whose major concern, in addition to other common complaints, was an escalating body weight gain that could not be stopped or reversed, regardless of what they ate. The vast majority of those patients were found to have low levels of free T3; when their free T3 level was increased as the result of taking desiccated thyroid, most began to see a gradual loss of body fat with an associated loss of body weight. Many of those patients began wearing clothes that they had not been able to wear for months or sometimes years. Of course, proper dietary habits were discussed and followed by all who were ultimately successful at losing body fat. It is unusual for a patient to complain of every symptom known to be associated with hypothyroidism; however, it is rather common for a patient to present with at least six-eight of those listed above.

No two patients are exactly alike and will present with different symptoms. Some patients complain of not having an appetite and are often thin. I realize that is the opposite of the typical patient stereotype, but simply illustrates how diverse the symptoms of hypothyroidism can be. There are other lesser common symptoms, but the above list provides a starting point. One can begin to comprehend my position that far too many drugs are used to treat the many symptoms of hypothyroidism and the cost is astronomical. The condition of hypothyroidism is being grossly under treated, but treating the symptoms of hypothyroidism has enriched pharmaceutical companies. Imagine a doctor diagnosing hypothyroidism and providing treatment by simply prescribing the appropriate dosage of desiccated thyroid. Also, imagine the vast amount of money saved if most doctors would simply exercise a modicum of common sense! Instead of prescribing one, two, or three anti-depressants, cholesterol-lowering agents, or high blood pressure medications, the hypothyroid patient with those conditions could realize an improvement in symptoms with thyroid replacement alone. The same holds true for many other symptoms listed above. Unfortunately, doctors have been conditioned and trained to treat symptoms, not the cause. As an example, we don't treat the cause of diabetes; we simply prescribe insulin or other drugs that facilitate the utilization of glucose. We don't treat the cause of high blood pressure, we treat the symptoms. In both of those examples, we must treat the symptoms because leaving either condition untreated is dangerous. What if we could treat the *cause* of those two common problems? Would that be welcomed by most doctors? I believe most doctors would be relieved to find a method to treat the cause of those two conditions instead of continuing to treat the symptoms. So why do doctors continue to treat the symptoms of hypothyroidism with various drugs while ignoring the actual hypothyroidism condition itself? In reference to my two examples of conditions for which we treat symptoms, I am not saying that both diabetes and hypertension always result from hypothyroidism. However, it is certainly logical to treat an underlying hypothyroid condition, if present, to determine its effect upon the course of either condition.

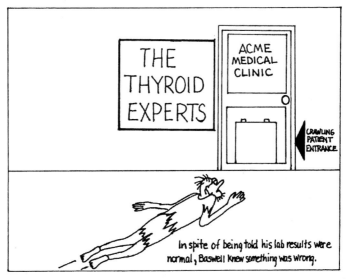

In spite of being told his lab results were normal, Baswell knew something was wrong.

Regardless of the symptoms, most doctors order standard tests including the TSH (Thyroid Stimulating Hormone) test, free T4 and T3 uptake. The TSH test is supposedly the "gold standard" test to diagnose hypo- or hyperthyroidism. It is also the test most doctors use to follow patients who are taking a thyroid supplement. A patient may have just enough energy to get out of the bed and drive to the doctor's office because their thyroid function is so low, but if the TSH test is considered in the normal range, it's as if the switch for common sense gets turned off with most doctors.

Please understand that doctors do that not because they are bad people who don't care, it's simply a matter of having been trained improperly and accepting propaganda as the truth! A patient can have a low TSH test and still be in need of thyroid supplementation.[10] Over ninety-five percent of patients with an undetectable TSH have a normal or low thyroid function.[11] [12]TSH is a hormone secreted by the pituitary gland and can be affected by medications, diseases, and pollutants. In other words, factors other than T4 can affect TSH levels. When the level of T4 is low, the TSH is usually elevated, and if it is elevated above what is currently considered the normal limit, the doctor may prescribe thyroid supplementation. The TSH is determined by the release of another hormone called Thyroid Releasing Hormone (TRH). It is released by an area of the brain called the hypothalamus, primarily in response to the level of free T4 that circulates in the blood stream. So when TRH signals the pituitary to secrete more TSH in response to low T4 in the blood, then the thyroid attempts to secrete more T4. The only problem is that T4 is not a very active molecule as indicated before. T4 is a thyroglobulin molecule that contains four atoms of iodine. Iodine is of major importance to the thyroid gland, but what many doctors do not understand is that iodine is important to the billions of other cells in the human body. T4 then undergoes a chemical change whereby one atom of iodine is removed resulting in the formation of T3, the major thyroid hormone. One would think that the molecule with more iodine is more important, but that is not the case! It is important to understand what I previously mentioned: **T3 is four to five times more potent than T4** and it is the hormone that will determine whether or not a patient is hypothyroid. It is T3 in the free state that is important! It is only the free portion of T3 that can bind to the specific T3 receptor site, causing the cell to react and create energy. Free T4 also binds, but it is not nearly as important. When the molecule is bound to a protein in order to be transported throughout the circulatory system, it can't attach to a receptor site. As a result, important and necessary chemical reactions do not take place. The hormone must be in the free state in order to bind at its receptor site. As indicated earlier, doctors test free T4, TSH, and T3 uptake. T3 uptake is an inverse measure of total T3, not free T3. That is why low thyroid function is missed so frequently. The TSH, free T4, and T3 uptake can all be normal in a person in dire need of thyroid supplementation. Most doctors treat the laboratory results and not the patient! That is partially because they don't know to order the correct test, nor do they know the *optimal value* of the free T3 test even if they were to order it. The normal values listed by laboratories for the free T3 are not what I have found to be the optimal values. To the contrary, the lower half of the "normal" range for free T3 is actually abnormal and consistent with a diagnosis of hypothyroidism. It is beyond the scope of this chapter to explain why this has happened and why this major error has continued to be maintained as being accurate. The short version is that laboratories have never considered the many factors involved in creating a population with an alarmingly high incidence of hypo-thyroidism. As a result, the normal ranges are simply not correct. In addition, doctors of today do not properly consider the patient's symptoms and complaints; they depend, instead, upon misleading lab studies. Again, this oversight is due primarily to the way doctors are trained and based upon what they don't know.

I have treated many patients who came to my office already taking the *synthetic version* of T4 (Synthroid®, Unithroid®, or Levoxyl®). Most were still having symptoms of hypo-thyroidism, but their doctors refused to increase the dose because their TSH was depressed. The literature is very clear in this regard and has indicated that patients are able to achieve optimal function and a feeling of well-being with a suppressed TSH.[13] Most doctors are not aware that published studies about this subject exist and continue to withhold thyroid as the result of a low TSH. I instruct all suspected hypothyroid patients to record their under arm (axillary) resting temperatures—before arising in the morning—and always obtain a free T3 laboratory study. In the vast majority of cases, their free T3 is extremely low (below optimal range), as are their resting axillary temperatures. For those already taking a synthetic T4 replacement, I typically change their thyroid replacement to *desiccated thyroid* and stop the synthetic variety of T4. I continue to monitor the free T3 and the body temperature. **A very high percentage of those patients typically begin to show improvement during the very first week.** They were all being treated by other doctors for hypothyroidism, but the fallacy of testing the TSH and treating with synthetic T4 resulted in most patients continuing to suffer the ill effects of hypothyroidism. There is no absolute conversion table when switching a patient from synthetic T4 to desiccated thyroid, but I typically replace fifty to sixty micrograms of synthetic T4 with one grain (60-65 milligrams) of desiccated thyroid.

The thyroid hormones major function is to stimulate mitochondrial activity. Proper mitochondrial activity regulates the body temperature, so it follows that recording body temperature would be a logical way to determine the level of thyroid function even without a test. Indeed, that is correct, as measuring body temperature is more accurate than any test yet devised. Since the extremity temperatures decrease before the core temperature decreases, it is advisable to obtain temperatures under the arm three mornings in a row before arising. Those mornings can be random for anyone except menstruating women who should take their temperatures on the second, third, and fourth morning of their period. The temperature under the arm is always less than an oral or rectal temperature and should be in the range of 97.8 to 98.2 degrees Fahrenheit. For those just starting thyroid supplementation, it takes several weeks for the temperature to rise to the acceptable range.

Dr. Broda Barnes was a brilliant endocrinologist who wrote a number of books about the thyroid in the 1970s. His ideas and commentary upon his research are just as good today as the day it was written. Dr. Barnes died in 1988 at the age of eighty-two, but his ideas and teachings are still ahead of the vast majority of his present day colleagues in endocrinology. Dr. Barnes was a proponent of obtaining axillary temperatures instead of the commonly accepted traditional laboratory tests. He also went into great detail about why this country would reach a point at which hypo-thyroidism would become an epidemic. He warned us and now the epidemic is here.

Unfortunately, again because of training and misinformation, most doctors will only prescribe synthetic thyroxine (T4). The makers of Synthroid engaged in a well-designed but misleading marketing campaign for many years. It appeared to me that their strategy was to give false information about their chief competitor (desiccated thyroid) in an attempt to gain a greater share of the thyroid supplement business. The campaign was very successful to the misfortune of many patients. Most doctors don't understand that they have been duped into believing that synthetic T4 is superior and even today continue prescribing it to the exclusion of the natural desiccated (dried) thyroid. Even the author of the chapter on thyroid in *Harrison's Textbook of Medicine*[14] indicates that he prefers the synthetic variety of T4 for the treatment of hypothyroidism. It is truly amazing what learned people will believe and repeat, regardless of the scientific basis. I know what doctors learn because I learned the same things and heard the same false stories.

It is not logical to treat patients with synthetic T4 exclusively. First, as I indicated before, T4 is a relatively unimportant hormone other than its ability to cross the blood-brain barrier to assist in the thought process, concentration, and memory. It stands to reason that patients should also be given a formula that also contains the much more important hormone, T3. One of the most important reasons for that is because there are many patients who have an impairment of converting T4 into T3 in the liver, kidneys, and other peripheral tissues. For a patient with conversion impairment who is only taking synthetic T4, that patient will remain hypothyroid—in spite of lab studies indicating otherwise—because their T3 levels will remain low. As alluded to earlier, many doctors seem to have left their common sense elsewhere when considering the diagnosis and treatment of hypothyroidism.

There are reasons why a patient has hypothyroidism. First, the thyroid gland itself may not be secreting sufficient hormone; but even more common and as noted above, the conversion of T4 to T3 may be impaired. It is not logical to prescribe additional T4 to a patient and expect an already compromised system to begin working properly and efficiently. If the patient has an impaired conversion mechanism, what will additional synthetic T4 actually accomplish? The answer is nothing! That is the very reason why T3 (contained in desiccated thyroid) must be given in all cases.

As noted, I have treated many patients that came to my office because their doctors refused to treat them with anything other than synthetic T4. In most cases, the patients still exhibited signs of hypothyroidism, but their doctors continued to get a TSH test that said they were normal. When I changed their prescription to a desiccated thyroid preparation containing T4, T3, and intrinsic factors that facilitate the action of both hormones, the vast majority of patients showed improvement. I have also had the experience of my patients seeing other doctors for unrelated problems during which time a TSH test was done. A number of my patients were told that their TSH was "dangerously" low because they were being "overdosed." Furthermore, many were advised to either reduce their dosage of desiccated thyroid or change to synthetic T4. The question always occurred to me, what danger were the patients in and why did they believe those patients to be overdosed? In all cases, the patients' resting pulse rates were normal and that is one of the major factors for determining the dosage for patients taking thyroid supplementation. Almost without exception, those patients had seen an increase of their body temperatures and had seen improvement of their initial symptoms. It is fortunate that patients still have a choice of remaining healthy by insuring proper thyroid levels; otherwise, they would be at the mercy of those whose practice is based upon myth and misinformation. It is simply illogical to reduce thyroid dosage in a patient who is improving and has a normal pulse. I typically prescribe desiccated thyroid simply because it works better and it avoids problems with those patients who have difficulty converting T4 to T3. Desiccated thyroid is derived from a porcine (pig) source, as the hormones are virtually identical to human thyroid hormones.

Another myth that seems to have been accepted in medical circles is that a low TSH can cause osteoporosis. That myth was based upon studies performed on menopausal females who were taking thyroid preparations.[15] When one takes a thyroid supplement, the TSH will decrease if the hypothalamus and pituitary are functioning properly. That is the way the thyroid feedback mechanism is supposed to work, but doctors seem to forget that most important fact. I am never surprised when my patients are tested by another doctor and a low TSH is found. I expect a low TSH in a patient who is taking a thyroid supplement; it is normal! Osteoporosis was found in many females that had depressed TSH when taking a thyroid preparation. However, their osteoporosis resulted from not taking sufficient estrogen, progesterone, and testosterone. The TSH had **nothing** to do with bone loss![16] [17] [18] [19] [20] Regardless, that myth has continued to be perpetrated within the medical community and other doctors have actually repeated that myth to my patients!

There are also patients who have what is referred to as "Type II" hypothyroidism. In that condition, the patient must supplement with more than the typical amount of thyroid and the level of free T3 can become very elevated. The reason for the condition is because the cell receptor sites for the thyroid hormone become sluggish and do not bind the hormone as readily as they should. It is otherwise referred to as thyroid hormone resistance. As a result, the level of hormone must be raised in order to make more hormones available at the receptor sites. Of course, the under arm temperatures and pulse/blood pressure are monitored until the optimal dose is determined. Periodic testing of free T3 is also performed. Entire books have been written about the subject of hypothyroidism alone. If the reader desires additional information about the subject, I would highly recommend the following books: *Hypothyroidism, the Unsuspected Illness* by Dr. Broda Barnes and *Hypothyroidism, Type 2, The Epidemic* by Dr. Mark Starr.

Another very important factor to consider is that many Americans are iodine deficient. This is particularly true for those living inland away from the seashore. Even those living near the seashore may be iodine deficient depending upon their diet. **Iodine is an important trace mineral that is necessary for proper cellular function**. This is the point at which many doctors lose sight of the importance of iodine. We know that iodine is of extreme importance to the thyroid since it is the component responsible for activation of a thyroglobulin molecule. As indicated earlier, T3 is much more active and potent than T4. Regardless of that fact, it becomes obvious that iodine deficiency can create a serious problem for the thyroid gland. Furthermore, much more iodine is needed by the body since the thyroid is not the only system that relies upon iodine for proper functioning.[21] A number of faulty studies have been performed that have misled doctors into believing that the body does not need as much iodine as it actually does.[22] In addition, they (doctors) have been led to believe by self appointed "experts" that iodine supplementation, above the level they suggest, can cause problems leading to iodism (toxicity to iodine). That's where fact and fiction begin to get confused.

What are the real problems caused by taking too much iodine and how much is too much? In order to understand the real issues and get factual answers, one must look at historical facts. Iodine is involved in a variety of vital functions in the human body other than the thyroid. It is a strong antioxidant, a bacteriocidal/virocidal (germ and virus killing) agent and free radical scavenger. It also stimulates optimum function of the immune system. A number of studies have shown that adequate (fifty to one hundred times the recommended daily allowance) intake of iodine is associated with a significantly lesser risk of breast cancer, polycystic ovary syndrome, and fibrocystic breast disease. In countries such as Japan, where the ingestion of iodine averages over 200 times the recommended dietary allowance (RDA), the incidence of breast cancer, fibrocystic breast disease, and polycystic ovary syndrome is virtually non-existent. Interestingly, Japanese people, consuming the typical diet rich in iodine, don't show any signs or symptoms of iodism (too much iodine). The symptoms of iodism are such things as a skin rash, metallic taste, painful teeth and gums, head congestion similar to symptoms of the common cold, and headaches. As the result of faulty misleading studies, many physicians have also been taught that one of the major effects of being exposed to too much iodine is hyperthyroidism with its attendant high pulse rate, increased blood pressure, headaches, anxiety and weight loss. That is very rare. After practicing medicine for over thirty-three years in four states, I have yet to see a single case! I have treated hundreds of patients with thyroid issues for the last twenty years and one would think I would have encountered at least one patient with iodism during that time. While it is possible that it occurs, it is extremely rare and when and if it does happen, probably involves factors other than iodine.

Studies about iodism have been faulty at best and contrived at worst. To say the studies are faulty simply means that most study designers did not adhere to scientific principles and many seem to have had a preconceived result in mind before the study was undertaken. That is simply intellectual dishonesty! The same type of people who perpetrated the myth about the earth being flat in the middle ages are very similar to the same types who perpetuate myths about iodine. Neither group wished to be confused by scientific facts. Those promoting the flat earth theory were primarily religious zealots that used their position and influence to maintain control, and with that, wealth and power. You may ask, what does this have to do with doctors and others who continue the war against iodine? Present day pseudo-scientists who continue the iodine myth are typically those in positions of influence and control. As the old saying goes, "The more things change, the more they stay the same." It is interesting how similar the close-minded of today are so similar to those with the same intellectually dishonest mindset from hundreds of years ago. What motivated the people in the past continues to motivate them today. Of course, there will always be the ignorant that perpetuate myths simply because they know no better, but many others remain entrenched because of money, control, and power. They are causing immeasurable problems because the value of iodine is vastly underestimated due to their continuing support of the iodine myth.

Many of you reading this will recognize the name Joseph Goebbels from reading the history of the Nazi regime and how they came to power in the 1930s. Goebbels was the Nazi Minister of Public Enlightenment and Propaganda during the Third Reich. He was a genius and his primary expertise was to have people believe outright lies. He said:

> If you tell a lie big enough and keep repeating it, people will eventually come to believe it. The lie can be maintained only for such time as the State can shield the people from the political, economic, and/or military [health] consequences of the lie. It thus becomes vitally important for the State [medical establishment] to use all of its powers to repress dissent, for the truth is the mortal enemy of the lie, and thus by extension, the truth is the greatest enemy of the State [self proclaimed experts in medicine].[23]

The appropriate substitutions were inserted to illustrate how this premise from over seventy years ago applies to present day medicine. It seems to me, the same premise used so well by Goebbels is being expertly used by those in positions of influence and power in the medical arena. When hypothyroid patients are under treated or not treated at all, the result is a patient population with myriad symptoms. Since most physicians fail to treat the underlying problem, the only things left to treat are the symptoms; drug companies are ready and willing to manufacture drugs in order to treat symptoms and reap the profits as a result. A similar scenario exists with iodine supplementation. That does not mean that your doctor is knowingly involved. On the contrary, as with other people, most doctors believe the lies they have been told, and it is now common in many areas of medicine for doctors to adhere to concepts that are based upon myths and misinformation. In other words, many doctors have become victims of a confidence game. The same concept espoused by Joseph Goebbels is alive and well in some aspects of present-day medicine. If one follows the money trail, it starts to become clear who and what is behind this continuing scam. I suppose one could start by watching those that complain the most when faced with facts that disagree with some of the currently accepted concepts.

When a person does not receive the necessary daily intake of iodine, the potential of developing health problems is significantly increased. The most obvious problem occurs with the thyroid gland, as it needs iodine to manufacture the hormones T3 and T4. When the thyroid becomes stressed because of the unavailability of iodine, it begins to compensate by enlarging **(goiter)** in an attempt to make more hormone. Other thyroid issues can also occur as a direct consequence of too little iodine. Thyroiditis (Hashimoto's) is another issue characterized by an inflammatory process wherein the body makes antibodies against its own thyroid that results in hypothyroidism. Others develop hyper-thyroidism, and the close-minded or self-serving would have everyone believe that it is heresy to treat those patients with iodine. In the past, when doctors actually examined and listened to patients, over ninety percent of hyperthyroid patients were successfully treated with iodine alone. It is ironic that doctors of today seem to have not learned anything from their very astute and competent colleagues from the past.

Lack of iodine also affects many other organ systems. For example, studies have been completed that have shown the benefit of iodine in preventing breast cancer, fibrocystic breast disease, and polycystic ovary syndrome just to name a few.[24] [25] [26] One would think that this information would be exciting news to those who write the textbooks and train new doctors; however, it has been suppressed by the same pseudo-scientists. One would also think the people raising money for the fight against breast cancer would be ecstatic about the studies showing the link between adequate intake of iodine and the reduction in the incidence of breast cancer. Suppose we were able to implement proper dosing of iodine and the incidence of breast cancer decreased to the same extent as in Japan. The urgency of finding a "cure" would diminish. I would never suggest that we should cease trying to find a cure for those who have breast cancer; but again, as the old saying goes, "An ounce of prevention is worth a pound of cure." Not only would the fundraising efforts for breast cancer be affected, but all the other problems brought about as the result of inadequate iodine intake would also lessen. If the incidence of problems related to inadequate iodine intake diminished, the need for treatment for those problems would become less as well. As you can begin to see, much of this issue revolves around economics, so one must ask the question about who benefits by perpetrating the continuing myths about iodine. The answer to that question should be quite obvious. It is comprised of those individuals and companies that profit by treating the many conditions that could be prevented by the proper intake of iodine.

I want to stress again that most doctors are genuinely concerned about their patients' health and truly attempt to offer the best care possible. However, the care they offer is directly related to their source and level of knowledge. If their knowledge is lacking, regardless of the reason, the diagnostic and treatment recommendations will be lacking as well. A person's well-being and health should be taken very seriously, and for that reason, it's advisable for patients to become proactive. In that regard, it is best to ask pertinent questions and, by all means, get proper answers. If a doctor refuses to discuss matters important to your health, then it's advisable to find a doctor who will discuss those issues. Avoid doctors who are hesitant to prescribe iodine because they are victims of propaganda and have chosen to remain misinformed. Also, avoid doctors who are reluctant or refuse to treat hypothyroidism with anything other than synthetic T4. They have been taken in by a slick marketing program and don't know that they have been scammed! Again, they are victims of lies perpetrated by those who benefit from perpetuating that same misinformation.

If you have symptoms that are consistent with those typically seen with hypothyroidism, take your resting under arm temperatures before arising. If the temperature is sub-optimal, report this to your doctor. If your doctor ignores your report or ridicules you and insists on testing your TSH instead of your free T3, it's advisable to find another doctor who is more knowledgeable. Doctors are human and humans make mistakes by believing lies stated as the truth. If a doctor doesn't know the answers to the questions a patient may ask, it is my advice to provide them the opportunity to learn more about the subject at hand. It is not the responsibility of patients to educate their doctors, but that's an individual issue that is made much more palatable when their doctor is willing to learn. If a doctor refuses to learn or scoffs at logical questions, it might be in the best interest of the patient to locate a more open-minded, science-based doctor because it's what your doctor doesn't know that can hurt you.

Notes

[1] Gull, W.W., "On cretinoid state supervening in adult life in women." *Trans Clin Soc Long*, 1874; 7:180-185.

[2] Murray, GR, "Note on the treatment of myxedema by hypodermic injections of an extract of the thyroid gland of a sheep." *BMJ*, 1891;2:796-797.

[3] MacKenzie, HW, "A case of myxedema treated with great benefit by feeding with fresh thyroid glands." *BMJ*, 1892;2:940.

[4] Fox, EL, "A case of myxoedema treated by taking extract of thyroid by mouth."*BMJ*, 1892;2:941.

[5] Baumann,E, "Ueber dasa normale Vorkommen Von Jodim Thierkorper." *Hoppe-Seylers A Physic Chem*, 1895;21:329-330.

[6] Kendall, EC, "the isolation in crystalline form of the compound which occurs in the thyroid: its chemical nature and physiologic activity." *JAMA*, 1915;64:2042-2043.

[7] Harrington, DR et al, "Thyroxine III, Constitution and synthesis of thyroxine." *Bio Chem J*, 1927;21:169-183.

[8] Chalmers,J.R. et al, "The synthesis of thyroxine and related substances. Part V. A synthesis of L-thyroxine from L-tyrosine." *J Chem Soc*, 1949:3424-3433.

[9] Gross, J et al, "The identification of 3:5:3'-:-triiodothyronine in human plasma." *Lancet*, 1952; 1:439-441.

[10] Igoe, D et al, *Journal of Medical Science*, Dec. 1992.

[11] Wheatley, T et al, *Annals of Clinical Biochemistry*, Sept. 1987.

[12] Allen, KR et al, *Annals of Clinical Biochemistry*, Sept. 1985.

[13] Ridgway, C et al, Clinical Endocrinology, Nov. 1980.

[14] *Harrison's Textbook of Medicine*, 12th edition, 1991, McGraw-Hill, New York.

[15] Toft, AD et al, *British Medical Journal*, May, 2003.

[16] Brokken, LS et al, *Journal of Clinical Endocrinology Metabolism*, Oct. 2001.

[17] Toth, M et al, *British Medical Journal*, May, 1987.

[18] Rachedi, F, *Press Med.* February, 1999.

[19] Fujiyama, K et al, *Thyroid*, February, 1995.

[20] Grant, DJ et al, *Clinical Endocrinology*, November, 1993.

[21] Abraham, G et al, "orthoiodosupplementation: Iodine Sufficiency of the whole human body." *The Original Internist*, 2002; 9(4):30-41.

[22] Wolff, J & Chaikoff, I, "Plasma inorganic iodide as a homeostatic regulator of thyroid function." J Biol Chem, 1948; 174:555-564.

[23] Evans, RJ, *The Third Reich in Power*, 2005.

[24] Finley, J & Bogardus, G, "Breast Cancer and thyroid disease." Quart Rev Surg Obstet Gynec, 1960; 17:139-147.

25 Thomas, BS et al, "Thyroid function in early breast disease." Europ J Cancer Clin Oncol, 1983; 19:1213-1219.

26 Wiseman, R, "Breast cancer hypothesis: a single cause for the majority of cases." J Epid Comm Health, 2000; 54: 851-858.

2

ANDROPAUSE

I know many of the men reading this have laughed and made jokes about their wife, grandmother, or mother going through "the change" (menopause). The joking occurred because of the abrupt and noticeable change in behavior of the lady involved. Even though it was attributed to hysteria, or other erroneous reasons, we now know why the female's relative behavior changed, or why they complained of "hot flashes" or night sweats, even if the outside temperature was low. Many men believed that menopausal women were exaggerating and poked fun as a result. Now that we understand the symptoms are real and quite common, we have lessened the tendency to joke, and simply accept it as a part of the aging process when a female reaches the age when the ovaries stop functioning after the child bearing years. Not only are the ovaries necessary for producing eggs (ova) which may be fertilized resulting in pregnancy, but the cessation of their activity results in the lowering of necessary hormones. The decline in hormones is manifested in the female by a number of symptoms: hot flashes, night sweats, and mood swings are all very common symptoms. All women have to go through the process, and once men realize that they also go through a similar phenomenon, it ceases to be so funny.

As in women, nature has a method of removing men from the breeding pool. However, that's only the tip of the iceberg as male menopause (andropause) has many health risks associated with it as well.[1] [2] The term "andropause" is derived from the Greek words "andro" (male) and "pausis" (stop). It wasn't a term that was accepted in medicine until the 1940s, and many doctors today continue to be non-accepting, regardless of the wealth of scientific evidence that proves its existence. The main hormone that determines when a male reaches andropause is testosterone; that, in turn, depends on what is being produced by his body. It is natural and genetically determined for a man to **gradually** produce less and less testosterone. As a result, the symptoms appear less suddenly in men than menopausal symptoms appear in women. Testosterone, for the most part, is produced by the testicles in response to another hormone, luteinizing hormone (LH) which is released by a part of the brain known as the pituitary. The pituitary, in turn, is controlled by hormones released by a part of the brain known as the hypothalamus. With aging, men gradually produce less testosterone year by year, and it surprises most to learn that this gradual decline begins in the mid-twenties. The primary reason this phenomenon occurs (hypogonadism) is because the testicles become less responsive to luteinizing hormone (LH), released by the pituitary. In other cases, pituitary production of LH is impaired, and its needed stimulus for the testes is lost. There are a number of drugs that can also contribute to andropause/hypogonadism, such as some diuretics, SSRIs, anti-fungals, major tranquillizers, statins, anti-convulsants, opioids, anti-convulsants, drugs to prevent hair growth by blocking formation of DHT, chemotherapy, cimetadine, chronic antihistamine use, corticosteroids, and some of the newer sleep meds such as Roserem® and Lunesta®. Hypothyroidism can also result in symptoms of andropause. The symptoms can be reversed in these instances by stopping the drug being taken, and correcting hypothyroidism, if this is an issue. Many of the symptoms associated with having to take the above noted drugs tend to improve when hormone optimization is undertaken. In those cases, the drugs may not be necessary any longer, but that is an individualized issue and has to be dealt with on a case-by-case basis. In most men, the andropause process is so gradual that many don't recognize the symptoms and just begin to feel that they are getting "old." The situation is made worse because their doctor may be telling them the same thing, **"You're just getting old,"** as if the male patients didn't already know that! If one hears that response from any doctor, it would probably be in their best interest to look elsewhere for medical help because none will be forthcoming from that type doctor. Of course, they are getting older, that's an inescapable fact, but the news is **something can be done about it!**

Regardless of the genetic cards one is dealt, more and more men are realizing that something can be done to offset the negative effects of declining levels of testosterone, but the process of education for the public and the medical profession has been rather slow and inefficient. One of the main factors, resulting in such an obsolete approach to this problem, has been that most doctors are not aware of the facts about the aging process and the importance of maintaining proper hormonal balance. That goes back again to the lack of, or improper training in the medical training systems. What is being taught takes many years to change, in spite of evidence to the contrary. As a result, it is the responsibility of every doctor to self-educate about this important subject. Quite frankly, the field of endocrinology (medical specialty focusing on hormones and disorders of endocrine glands) should have a monopoly on this interesting and vitally important area, but such is not the case. As a matter of fact, some of the major opponents of optimal hormonal balance are specialists in endocrinology. On the other hand, there are a few endocrinologists that have recognized the deficiencies of how and what they have been taught and have chosen to further their knowledge in this often misunderstood arena. Some of the most astute physicians I know are endocrinologists. They are the individuals that have furthered their knowledge in this remarkable field by analyzing some of the questionable, but accepted, standards of care. Why do most endocrinologists remain years behind in this constantly changing and evolving field? It has been my observation that many within this specialty possess very little scientific curiosity, particularly regarding concepts not taught during their residency training.

That lack of intellectual and scientific curiosity seems to be inherent. Even when exposed to undisputable scientific facts that differ with the dogma so ingrained within their specialty, they remain steadfast in their effort to stall progress. When politics and blind adherence to dogma and protocol are chosen over science, a dangerous situation can result that will adversely affect patients who do not receive appropriate care. For additional information about this situation, please review the chapter on hypothyroidism.

How does a male know when he is a candidate for testosterone replacement? There are a number of symptoms consistent with low testosterone, and the one most men concern themselves with is the subject of libido (sex drive). There are a number of other signs, but this is the one that concerns most men as it strikes at their masculinity and is perceived in a very personal manner. Of course that is understandable, but there are other important factors associated with low levels of testosterone, which most men, and many doctors, don't recognize. For example, many of my female patients speak to me about their spouses or boyfriends, and whether or not they should be evaluated. I hear about myriad symptoms such as low energy, depression, loss of sex drive, lack of stamina, weight gain, loss of muscle mass, loss of strength, and moodiness.

All the above are symptoms of low testosterone, but the most important factor is the one that is never mentioned and unknown to most doctors. Testosterone has a protective effect on the cardiovascular system. In other words, higher levels of testosterone protect the heart and brain. Dr. Jens Moller, a Danish physician, studied the effects of testosterone in men for over thirty years.[3] Studies are ongoing in Denmark about this very subject and the results have been very convincing and conclusive, that testosterone has this very important cardiovascular protective effect. Essentially, the researchers found that lower levels of testosterone are associated with a higher incidence of heart disease, while higher levels of testosterone are associated with a lower incidence. In Europe, heart disease and vascular disease are frequently treated with testosterone. Not only are the results experience oriented, but scientific studies have now shown why this phenomenon occurs. Cells exist within the lining of arteries that are referred to as "foam cells." Higher levels of testosterone prevent enlargement of foam cells and they remain relatively dormant and insignificant. However, when testosterone levels decline, as a man ages or for any other reason, control over the growth of foam cells is lost. As foam cells enlarge, they often rupture through the interior of an artery wall into the lumen (opening). When that takes place, it establishes a site favorable for plaque formation which typically gets progressively larger with the passage of time. Plaque is caused when calcium and cholesterol accumulate at one or more locations in an artery. Because cholesterol becomes part of the plaque, many people, including doctors, believe that heart attacks and strokes are caused by high cholesterol. In truth, cholesterol is not the villain it has been portrayed to be. Without the site of formation, cholesterol is a relatively harmless, but necessary substance. If the plaque gets too large, then it can block blood flow. If that happens, a heart attack or stroke can occur. One would think that doctors and government bureaucrats would be interested in reducing the incidence of heart disease and stroke in this country. So why has testosterone treatment not been recognized as being able to treat these conditions? The answer is multi-faceted, but revolves around ignorance of the facts and an unwillingness to learn. In this country, medical students are taught to never give testosterone to anyone with documented atherosclerotic vascular disease (hardening of the arteries). The correct information is available, backed by a number of properly designed studies that refute this error. So why is it being withheld?

One problem arises when studies with a faulty design are taken seriously enough to be published. A recent study was published in the July 8, 2010 issue of the prestigious *New*

England Journal of Medicine entitled, "Adverse events associated with testosterone administration."[4] The subjects of the study were men with a median age of seventy-four, most had pre-existing heart disease, did not exercise, were cigarette smokers, and were overweight. After gaining an improvement in strength as the result of being administered testosterone, these same men were asked to perform exercises to demonstrate strength gains. The men receiving testosterone showed a higher incidence of heart problems than those not taking testosterone. Is it truly surprising that these men sustained a higher incidence of heart related issues in view of their history? They were compared to a similar group of men who were not given testosterone and, in spite of all the other variables, the authors of the study concluded that testosterone was the culprit! The men not taking testosterone did not have any measurable strength gains and were not able to perform similarly to the control group. This is a prime example of having a pre-conceived notion prior to a study being undertaken. The only thing proven by the study was to be cautious in administering testosterone to men with a median age of seventy-four, who are obese, smokers, have heart disease, and do not exercise. This is one of the reasons why this life saving hormone continues to be maligned. As evidenced by this article, it even happens at prestigious institutions in which we should have the utmost faith. When my patients are exposed to the information about the protective effects of testosterone, most are quite surprised since they had never heard this from another doctor. Once the majority of my patients learn the science-based facts, they typically become more proactive.

Testosterone is also important in maintaining healthy bones. Proper levels (optimal) help maintain proper mineralization and add to the strength of bones. When bones are stronger, they are much less likely to fracture with minimal trauma.

When most men become aware of the cardiovascular and skeletal protective effect of testosterone, they strive to never let their blood levels fall to previously accepted "normal" levels. That brings up the point of what doctors consider normal. As an example, if we were to study 1,000 men, age sixty, the average level would prove to be much lower than a sample of 1,000 men at twenty-five years of age. When a doctor tells a male patient over the age of forty-five that his levels are normal, what he/she is really saying is that compared to everyone else in that age group, their levels are about the same. Apparently it never occurs to most doctors that if everyone in a particular age group is low, then a low level will be considered "normal" as well. Normal does not mean that it's healthy, it's just a mathematical number computed from averages in a particular age group. This illustrates something very important and something lost in doctors' training programs. **Normal values do not necessarily mean "optimal."** Optimal levels of testosterone allow starved receptor sites to bind the testosterone molecule the way it is intended. Binding simply means that the testosterone attaches to a part of the cell that is made specifically for the purpose of binding with testosterone. When binding takes place, the cellular reaction, stimulated by testosterone, will then take place.

The effects of testosterone are many, but most men are concerned primarily with the libido (sex drive) effect. Since the time a male's body underwent puberty, the majority of men experienced the positive libido effect of testosterone because the body produces a high amount during, and just after, puberty. However and as previously mentioned, the amount of testosterone secreted begins to diminish gradually in the mid-twenties; so gradually, that many men do not recognize the impact until their symptoms are very apparent.

How is it determined that testosterone levels are not optimal? First of all, the symptoms alone typically help make a tentative diagnosis, but blood studies can verify the accuracy of that diagnosis. The total level of testosterone should be checked, but more importantly, it is the free level of testosterone that is more diagnostic. I also obtain a PSA (prostatic specific antigen), which measures a protein, secreted by the prostate, that is elevated with infection, inflammation, enlargement, and cancer. Luteinizing hormone (LH) and follicle stimulating hormones (FSH) should also be checked in many circumstances. Those are stimulating hormones secreted by the pituitary. LH, stimulates the Leidig cells of the testicles to secrete testosterone, and the importance of that test will be described. FSH or follicle-stimulating hormone is responsible for how much sperm a man produces in his Sertoli cells, which I check when a man expresses a desire to have children. I also check the level of estradiol (estrogen) as well, because elevated levels are not healthy, and interfere with how well testosterone works. Sex hormone binding globulin (SHBG) is also important because it measures the protein that binds free testosterone and transports it through the blood to target cells. If SHBG is too high, then it binds too much free testosterone and prevents it from binding to receptor sites. As noted, free testosterone has to bind to specific cell receptors, otherwise it does not work. Therefore, a high SHBG is contrary to the proper attachment of free testosterone at receptor sites. Once the results of the studies are available to me, then I can make a determination of where the patient's levels fall in regard to what is optimal. As I indicated before, normal levels are typically not optimal.

When it is determined that testosterone levels are not optimal, there are a variety of ways to increase those levels in order to reach the optimal range. In men below fifty years of age, I have found that human chorionic gonadotropin (HCG) successfully stimulates many to produce enough testosterone of their own to bring them into the optimal range. It works by increasing levels of FSH and LH that, in turn, cause the production of more sperm and testosterone respectively. HCG typically doesn't work as well for those over the age of fifty, but there are always exceptions. I also use a preparation called clomiphene, that works in a manner similar to HCG by stimulating production of FSH and LH that can result in increased levels of both sperm and testosterone. HCG and clomiphene are the most reliable methods of increasing a male's sperm and testosterone, but only in men that are responsive. HCG is administered via a subcutaneous injection that is performed three days per week; the typical dose is 250-500 units. HCG can also be applied as a cream three times per week. Clomiphene is taken orally in the form of a capsule or tablet and is also prescribed three times per week or on alternative days if more convenient for the patient. The patient's laboratory values are checked again after six weeks to determine whether or not either was effective in increasing the patient's level of testosterone. If neither is effective, because of various reasons, then testosterone must then be supplemented.

I prefer to not give testosterone in a capsule, pill, or tablet form because it results in an extra step, involving absorption through the gastrointestinal tract and being metabolized by the liver. I never use any preparation containing methyl testosterone because that particular form of testosterone has been proven to be toxic and can cause many side effects. Some of the available scientific studies about testosterone used methyl testosterone, resulting in giving testosterone a bad name because of the toxicity of that particular form. Many doctors still don't recognize this very important fact and continue to remain overly cautious about this life restoring, and sometimes life-saving, hormone. When possible, I prefer to use bio-identical testosterone in a cream, gel, drops, sublingual (under the tongue) tablets, subcutaneous pellets, or lozenges. If a patient does not absorb adequately with the use of these methods, I will then consider subcutaneous (under the skin) injections of either testosterone cypionate or enanthate. By using any of these methods I suggest, all bypass the step of being absorbed through the intestine, and get directly into the blood stream by being absorbed through capillaries in the skin, mucous membranes, or subcutaneous tissues. The method chosen depends on the individual, but there can be problems with any of these methods mentioned. With sublingual drops, lozenges, creams, gels, or sublingual tablets, some people do not absorb them well, and their levels never reach the optimal range. If this happens, I prescribe injectable testosterone. In the past, testosterone was injected into the muscle, but it has been determined that it is more physiologic (mimics nature) to inject it under the skin.[5] I teach the patient to self-inject, which is actually fairly simple once a patient gives himself his first injection under my supervision. The problem associated with the injection method is obvious, and involves the patient's concern about needles. I have experience with patients who refused to inject themselves, and therefore, have no choice other than using the absorption method, via the subcutaneous tissue with a pellet, or under the tongue. The downside to the creams, gels, lozenges and drops is the fact that it has to be done twice daily. The half-life of testosterone is fairly short, making a once a day regimen inappropriate because the levels will fall from the optimal range before taking the next dose. Half-life is the term used to describe how long it takes to eliminate half the dose from the system. Pellets are effective and maintain optimal levels for about three to five months before having to be replaced. The problem arises if the wrong dose is implanted, making necessary changes quite difficult. For that reason, I have avoided recommending implantable pellets. Injections are given every six to seven days, depending upon the preparation and the laboratory values. Injectable testosterone has a greater half-life than creams, gels, or lozenges. In the past, men received testosterone injections once a month, but it's become apparent that neither the manufacturers, nor the physicians, considered the limited half-life of the preparation when dosing in that fashion. The typical response, when following that dosage schedule, was to create a high supraphysiologic (excessive) level of testosterone initially, followed by a decline to a sub-optimal range during the next few weeks. That resulted in a so-called "roller coaster effect." It is very unnatural, and will not provide the optimal benefits and effects of testosterone if dosed in that manner, but some doctors continue exactly that method, simply because that's how they were taught. The injections use a preparation of testosterone cypionate or enanthate. Neither are bioidentical, but the preparation is metabolized very easily, resulting in bio-identical testosterone being made available. It is the addition of a side chain on the molecule that results in the extended half-life of the preparation after injection.

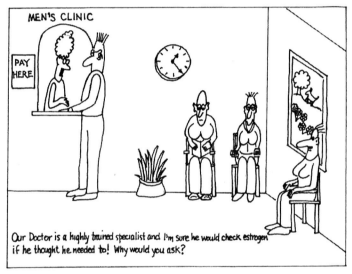

effects of testosterone if dosed in that manner, but some

Many feel that their problem is solved once they begin taking testosterone, but that is not always the case. The blood levels must be checked periodically to make certain the patient is staying in the optimal range. For example, I have seen patients who had been taking testosterone prescribed by other doctors, whose levels were far below optimal range because of infrequent dosing or inadequate dosage. Both the strength and frequency of dosage must be maintained in order to provide for levels in the optimal range. As I indicated earlier, I also monitor levels of estradiol (estrogen) and SHBG. If either of those increase beyond certain levels, the patient will experience problems, which typically cannot be solved by altering the dose of testosterone. Instead, medications are available to reduce levels of either substance. In men, estrogen is made from testosterone, primarily in the fatty tissues with the help of an "aromatase" enzyme. This process can only be counteracted with a preparation that blocks the enzyme from working. Excess estrogen can cause unwanted results with growth of breast tissue and the accumulation of fat deposits on the hips and thighs. Men who have greater degrees of abdominal fat tend to have greater degrees of testosterone to estrogen conversion, since much of the conversion takes place in the abdominal fat. This is the major reason why I advise men not to inject testosterone into the abdominal area. If estrogen levels increase, an aromatase inhibitor is prescribed and subsequent testing typically finds their estrogen back in the acceptable range. Some estrogen is good, but too little or too much is not. SHBG should also remain in the acceptable range as well. If it increases beyond that range, then problems can occur when too much testosterone binds to that protein. If there is not enough free testosterone available to bind to cell receptor sites, then it's the same as having too little testosterone, even though it is being supplemented. When the SHBG increases, it must be reduced, and there are only a couple of preparations that will cause that to happen. Once the prescription preparations are taken as directed, these levels typically fall, and the patient begins to experience all the good and healthy effects of optimal testosterone levels.

It typically takes about three to four weeks before a patient begins to appreciate the full benefits of testosterone replacement, provided the blood levels are in the optimal range and there's not too much estrogen or SHBG being created. I have treated many patients who came to my office for their second visit telling me that they felt great for two to three weeks, after which they began to notice a gradual decline. That's the time laboratory testing is most appropriate and I'm able to correct the problem of interference by estrogen or SHBG.

One question that I hear often is, "Do I have to take this the rest of my life?" Many people are brainwashed and don't understand that the replacement of hormones is not a short-term fix or something to be taken to cure an illness; to the contrary, it is a life-long process. Diminished hormones occur because the body is not producing enough of that hormone and never will again, simply because it's a natural process for those hormones to decline. If a patient decides to stop taking testosterone, then all body functions in regard to that hormone will decline to the suboptimal levels expected with lower levels. Essentially, the testosterone level will return to the pre-treatment level and body functions will continue to decline as long as the hormone levels remain in the sub-optimal range. If one truly wishes to optimize their health, then the prescribed hormone(s) should be taken for the remainder of their life.

What about side effects? As I indicated in another part of the book, I spend a great deal of time with my patients dispelling rumors about hormone replacement. Each hormone has its own set of questions, including those for testosterone. As an example, "Will it cause me to grow breasts?" It can and often does when the serum (blood) levels are not being checked, as with athletes or body builders who inject, or take anything and everything, without medical supervision. Growth of breast tissue can occur when levels of estrogen are allowed to increase beyond healthy levels. That is one of the reasons why the level of estrogen must be monitored.

Another question I hear often is, "Will testosterone cause shrinkage of the testicles and will it be permanent?" Yes, it can cause shrinkage, as it is the body's natural method of ensuring that we don't produce too much testosterone. When levels of testosterone are in the high normal or optimal range, part of the brain called the hypothalamus interprets those levels to mean that the testicles don't need to make more testosterone. The hypothalamus then doesn't release gonadotropin-releasing hormone (GnRH) that is necessary to signal the pituitary to release more LH and FSH. In turn, when LH and FSH are not released, the body is not stimulated to produce sperm and testosterone. When the testicles are not stimulated, they can decrease in size. However, shrinkage can be reversed or prevented by taking either clomiphene or HCG. A less viable option is to stop taking the testosterone. To the contrary, it is highly inadvisable to stop taking testosterone once it is started, simply because of its many health benefits and the known risks of low testosterone.

Another frequent question is "Will I become dependent on testosterone?" Testosterone is not a drug, it is a hormone that one's own body makes, but it just doesn't make enough to maintain optimal health after a certain age. You will not become dependent upon testosterone, but it is in your best interest to supplement it in order to gain the many health benefits.

"Does testosterone cause prostate cancer?" There is no evidence that testosterone causes prostate cancer. If that were true, then it would be the men with higher levels who get prostate cancer, and that would certainly include most males from puberty to their mid- to late-twenties. It's not the men with higher levels of testosterone that get prostate cancer; to the contrary, it is more commonly the group of men who have low levels of testosterone. It has been suggested that one of the contributing factors of prostate cancer, other than environmental contaminants, is estrogen from the conversion of testosterone, which predisposes men to prostate cancer.[6] [7] This is why it is vitally important for your doctor to check the hormone estradiol if you are taking testosterone supplementation. Estradiol is a cell proliferative hormone. If left unchecked, it can cause growth of breast tissue and fatty tissue in the hips and thighs. In women, it is the hormone that prepares the uterus for pregnancy by causing growth of endometrial tissue. In men, it can cause growth of prostate tissue with accompanying enlargement of the prostate. It has already been discussed that men make estrogen from testosterone, and that this tendency increases with age. As an example, I often see older men with very low levels of testosterone and high estrogen levels on their first visit.

"Will testosterone make me aggressive or antagonistic?" The answer to that depends on whether or not the person was aggressive or antagonistic in their younger years. If so, then testosterone will tend to bring back underlying personality traits. For most of my patients, testosterone tends to make them mellower and less moody. Most of the men who tend to get angry over trivial issues have lower levels of testosterone and that tendency is reduced once the levels increase.

"What if I stop taking testosterone?" If a patient stops taking something they need for optimal function, then their ability to function will return to essentially the same level they were before starting the testosterone. It typically takes between ten and fourteen days before the system returns to the pre-treatment levels. Of course, the problems that prompted them to start testosterone will also return, and they lose the cardiovascular and skeletal protection as well.

"Will it cause me to lose my hair?" There is a genetic predisposition for hair loss in certain men that is known as male pattern hair loss. The exact reason for the condition is not fully understood, but we know that a breakdown product of testosterone, Dihydrotestosterone (DHT), plays a role in accelerating the process. As a result, a number of prescription drugs are available that prevent the conversion of testosterone to DHT. According to many sources, and my personal observation of many male patients, the drugs do work to a certain extent by reducing the rate of hair loss. However, DHT is also an important hormone for stimulating the libido (sex drive). When DHT is lowered, the libido sometimes suffers as well. The names of drugs used for this purpose include Propecia®, Proscar®, Avodart®, and Minoxidil®. All can adversely affect the libido and sexual performance. As an alternative, I suggest a compound that is used in a shampoo that works locally at the hair follicle and does not absorb systemically to any significant degree. It contains a drug that blocks the conversion of testosterone to DHT, T3 thyroid hormone, and thymus extract. Because it is applied locally, it only blocks DHT where it can do the most damage, at the hair follicle.

"Will testosterone cause me to bulk up and become muscle bound?" Testosterone is a naturally occurring anabolic (building) hormone that will result in retention of muscle mass and an improvement in strength. Males who exercise routinely and are taking testosterone can see muscle growth and an improvement in their strength, similar to the same process seen in their youth. The harder they work, within reasonable limits, the more gains they will see. However, it will typically not result in excessive muscle growth and strength gains beyond that seen in their youth.

"Will testosterone cause my skin to breakout?" Some men experience acne when taking testosterone, but those patients are typically the same people who experienced acne problems during puberty. For those individuals with acne problems, they can be treated with a daily low dose of tetracycline.

"I'm going to have surgery and my doctor told me to stop taking all drugs." The key term in what the surgeon said was, stop taking all **DRUGS.** Hormones, including testosterone, **ARE NOT** drugs! The purpose for a surgeon telling a patient to stop taking drugs is simply to avoid any problems associated with drugs, which might interfere with the surgical process or the anesthesia provided. Maintaining optimal levels of hormones is important for stimulating the healing process and should be continued as directed. Keep in mind that **drugs** are chemicals foreign to the human metabolism. Bioidentical hormones are identical to hormones the human body manufactures naturally.

"Are there negative effects of testosterone when it is used properly?" The short answer to that question is no, but a small percentage of patients experience mild fluid retention that usually resolves after six to eight weeks. Some patients experience some flushing (redness) of the face and neck, but typically seen only in fair-skinned males whose levels exceed the optimal range. It also tends to diminish with time and/or the reducing of the dosage.

"Can I take too much testosterone?" Yes, one can take too much, which will result in the conversion to excessive estradiol. The other problem is that it can make testosterone receptor sites less responsive (down regulation of receptor sites). If this happens, many men, who are not under medical supervision, tend to increase their dose when, in fact, it is the opposite of what should be done. The dose of testosterone should actually be decreased, or stopped temporarily, in an effort to up-regulate the receptor sites.

"Is there an alternative to taking testosterone?" One may assume that the answer to that is a definite "no", but that is not necessarily the case. As noted previously, younger men, typically below the age of fifty, sometimes respond to HCG and/or clomiphene as they both increase the levels of FSH and LH. In turn, LH stimulates the testicles to produce and release more testosterone, while FSH stimulates the production of sperm. If the stimulation by either, or both, of those medications results in an optimum level of testosterone, then actual testosterone supplementation is not necessary. However, the response will eventually diminish, and testosterone will have to be supplemented at that time. For those who are only concerned about a diminishing sex drive and performance, a study revealed that Acetyl-L-carnitine and Propionyl-L-carnitine are as effective as testosterone for that purpose.[8] However, one shouldn't ignore the known protective effect of testosterone with regard to the heart, vascular system, and bones. Combining testosterone with those compounds is the best alternative, and provides the benefits of both.

In summary, all men go through a process (andropause), similar to menopause in women. Depending upon genetics, the process develops at different rates. Some younger men are affected earlier than most, and may begin to notice a decline as early as the fourth decade of life (thirties). Some older men are affected less than most, and don't begin to notice a decline until their fifties; but, eventually all men will be affected by andropause. Some physicians deny the importance of declining testosterone and focus on whether or not the patient remains in the normal laboratory range, while ignoring the many deleterious effects of low testosterone. The most obvious difference between men and women, in this regard, is that the reduction in the hormonal levels occurs on a much more gradual basis in men, but all symptoms can be reversed by adding testosterone supplementation, provided all other hormones are balanced as well. There is virtually no downside to supplementing with testosterone and the positive effects are many and significant.

Notes

[1] Traish, AM et al, "The dark side of testosterone deficiency:II. Type 2 diabetes and insulin resistance." *Journal of Androl* 2009; 30(1):23-32.

[2] Pike CJ et al, "Androgens, aging and Alzheimer's disease." *Endocrine*, April 2006; 20(2):233-241.

[3] Moller J. & Einfeldt H., "Testosterone Treatment for Cardiovascular Diseases." *Springer-Verlag*, Berlin,1984.

[4] Basaria, S. et al, "Adverse events associated with testosterone administration." *New England Journal of Medicine*, July 8, 2010; 363(2):109-122.

[5] Al-Futaisi AM et al, "Subcutaneous administration of testosterone. A pilot study report." *Saudi Med J.*, 2006 Dec. 27(12):1843-1846.

[6] Farnworth, WE, "Roles of estrogen and SHBG in prostate physiology. *Prostate*, Jan 1996; 28(1):17-23.

[7] *Scandinavian Journal of Urology and Nephrology.* March 1995; 29(1):65-68.

[8] Cavallini, G et al, "Carnitine vs androgen administration in the treatment of sexual dysfunction, depressed mood and fatigue associated with male aging." *Urology*, 2004; 641:641-646.

3

WOMEN AND HORMONES

Women have recognized and dealt with changes brought about as the result of declining hormones for many years. Of course, I'm referring to **menopause,** or the climacteric through which all women eventually proceed. In essence, it means the end of child bearing years, because ovulation ends as well. Certain levels of hormones are necessary in order to help ovaries to produce an egg (ovum), and when that declines, so does the ability to develop an egg that is viable and ready for fertilization. The proper cycling of hormones also readies the female's uterus for pregnancy. When the egg is not fertilized, the body then undergoes further changes due to hormonal fluctuations, resulting in the shedding of the endometrium, which is eliminated when the women undergo the monthly cycle known as the menses (period). Menopause also signals the end of the menses; for many women, that's a welcome relief, but for others, it results in a degree of sadness. Menopause is simply the way genetic programming removes women from the reproductive pool, but it certainly doesn't mean that life is over. It does mean that women must become proactive, as important health matters need to be considered.

The typical scenario of menopause commonly begins in the fifth decade (forties) of a female's life. The time of onset can vary, but it typically begins in that decade with the actual average age of their final period being around fifty-one years Western civilization.[1] There are a variety of menopausal symptoms, including scanty or irregular periods in women who had regular three to five day periods their entire productive life (from puberty to menopause). Early on, many women begin to feel "hot flashes" on an irregular basis, which become more frequent as time passes. Night sweats are another common feature that gradually becomes more prominent as the female proceeds further through the menopausal process. The hot flashes and night sweats are secondary to vasomotor instability, resulting from an imbalance between estrogen and progesterone. The beginning stages of menopause are referred to as perimenopause or premenopause. The beginning stage is variable in duration and different for every female. It can continue for two to three years or be as short as two to three months. Once a woman enters full menopause, the symptoms of perimenopause can many times intensify, signaling the further reduction of three sex hormones, estrogen, progesterone, and testosterone. The nuisance symptoms of hot flashes, night sweats, dry skin, atrophy of genitourinary tissue, irritability, lowered sex drive, anxiety, and depression may worsen, while other women have minimal symptoms.

In this day and age, with the vast exposure to estrogen-like compounds in our food and environment, it is wise for all women to begin testing their levels of sex hormones during their mid-thirties. Most women wait until they are experiencing obvious symptoms, such as hot flashes and night sweats, before consulting a doctor. It is more proactive and wiser to have baseline lab values available before symptoms begin. If a hormone imbalance is identified, it will alert the doctor and patient alike, so that it can be corrected, and the many negative consequences can be avoided.

When this inevitable change takes place, the majority of women rely upon the help of their gynecologist or family doctor. Unfortunately, many gynecologists and family doctors of today may not recognize the importance of only replacing a female's hormones with those that adapt best to her body because they are specific for the human female. Instead, and similar to physicians in other specialties, they have been misinformed and led to believe that chemical substitutes are just as good as the real thing. Nothing could be further from the truth, but you have to remember, it's what your doctor doesn't know that can hurt you. If a female complains of symptoms suggestive of menopause, her gynecologist or family doctor typically prescribes Premarin®. Why do they prescribe that particular preparation? For the same reasons listed in the preface to this book. The doctors who taught them taught them improperly because they didn't use science and logical thinking, instead allowing the pharmaceutical industry a self-serving voice. Most accepted the propaganda disseminated by pharmaceutical companies who profit from doctors prescribing their products. They prescribe Premarin because the manufacturing company has engaged, and continues to engage, in a successful marketing campaign. If your doctor prescribes Premarin, he/she has simply and most probably been taken in by marketing propaganda, and has become desensitized to the undeniable fact that bioidentical hormones are far superior. Bioidentical hormones have the exact molecular structure as those made by the human body. That is a very important concept to understand when critics compare bioidentical hormones to non-bioidentical substitutes made by drug companies. I have consulted with many female patients who actually believed that Premarin was a human estrogen combination, and did not know that the compound was derived from the urine of pregnant mares (horses). This widely used product has been around since 1942 and the FDA has yet to acknowledge all the different types of estrogen in the compound! While Premarin has some estrogen, which is the same as that found in humans, a number of the estrogens are unique to horses and have no known purpose in a human female. The company simply states that it's a "natural" conjugated estrogen compound. **It is "natural," but only for horses, not human beings!**

Women require only three forms of estrogen at receptor sites, regardless of their age and circumstances, and will never require any other type of estrogen. There are a number of metabolites of estrogen, but those are not involved in the receptor binding process and have no known physiological function. The physiologically pertinent estrogens are estradiol, estrone, and estriol. We know that Premarin has at least ten types of estrogen, and most of those are unique to horses. Why would any informed woman want to take a preparation that is intended for a horse? Would it be logical to use a Volkswagen part in a Ferrari? That's a big NO! It's simply not logical to use parts in a car that are not made for that car! So why do mechanics seem to understand the importance of using a correct component on cars, while doctors have been led to believe that prescribing correct hormones for women is less important? Why settle for questionable substitutes, particularly when bioidentical hormones are readily available? The human body should be provided the hormones that are identical to those made by the human body! The problem with Premarin revolves around the fact that prescribing physicians seemingly don't understand the basic premise that we should not be putting hormones in the human body that are intended for horses. Unbelievable as that sounds, it is true and can be verified by asking your doctor why he/she prefers Premarin. The answers will be revealing, but most will advise you that the product has been available for a long time and it's okay, or some answer similar in nature. In other words, they really don't know the difference and have no idea they have been led astray. The makers of Premarin seem to have escaped critical scrutiny for over sixty-five years![2] With the escalating incidence of cancer in this country, why take chances that are not necessary? Even current news stories indicate a breast cancer connection between using combination products containing conjugated horse estrogens and progestin's (progesterone chemical look-alikes).

Horse estrogens are used in a number of other brand-name products that your doctor may prescribe without adequate consideration. Because of that, it is important to read labels, package inserts, and other available information. If you find this somewhat disturbing, keep reading because the next example will cause you even more reason for concern. Even though your doctor may not be aware of the facts about

Premarin as opposed to bioidentical hormones, it does not necessarily mean that he/she doesn't have your best interests at heart. **Most doctors are truly good people and don't mean you any harm, but it's what they don't know that can hurt you.**

Another product, manufactured by the same pharmaceutical company, is called Prempro®. For many years a number of doctors and scientists had been contending that horse estrogens were probably not the best choice to use in human females and the alarm was also sounded against using another hormone look-alike called progestin. It looks and acts like progesterone, but it's a wolf in sheep's clothing. Many doctors questioned whether or not progestin's were causing avoidable problems in women, but the supporters of progestin always replied that there was no proof. As a result, a study was undertaken to look at the drug Prempro. Be aware that Prempro is a combination of horse estrogens (Premarin) and progestin, specifically, medroxyprogesterone acetate, which the company labels as MPA to make it sound acceptable. MPA is NOT progesterone and never will be, but it can be patented because it was developed in the laboratory. Specifically, Prempro is a combination of two things that should not, in my opinion, be given to women. However, because of marketing, gynecologists and family doctors continue to write perscriptions for this very questionable combination hormone replacement concoction.

As indicated, the Women's Health Initiative study was undertaken to determine and analyze the side effects of Prempro, but it was stopped short of its scheduled completion date because the bad effects were already becoming quite evident.[3] The study showed an increased incidence of cancer, dementia, heart attacks, and strokes in women taking Prempro. The results were published in 2002, and instead of performing their due diligence and understanding what the study was about, many women simply stopped taking "all" hormones. This problem was made worse because many doctors didn't understand the study results either and went along with the mass hysteria. It was actually very simple; the study was about a patented drug, Prempro! It was not about **bioidentical hormones that women need in order to achieve and maintain optimum health.** More recent misinformation has also been spread about "hormones" causing increased breast cancer rates. Again, what hormones? The latest study published in the *Journal of the American Medical Association (JAMA)* on Tuesday October 19, 2010, cited findings in women using the same preparation, Prempro! It begs the question as to why it remains on the market. The answer to that question should prompt doctors to look at many patented drugs in a very skeptical manner. Based upon scientific studies, we already know that Prempro increases risk for a number of very serious diseases, but the company is still selling it! You may ask yourself why your doctor doesn't know that. The answer is because they get most of their information from the company that manufactures the drug, who further justify prescribing it by telling doctors that all drugs have side effects. I believe many doctors are so misinformed that they truly don't recognize the tremendous difference between bioidentical hormones and chemicals. Accordingly, it is the responsibility of the patient to become proactive instead of being a statistic.

I often hear the following question from menopausal women, "Why should I take hormones if I'm not experiencing any symptoms?" The answer to that question involves dispelling another myth. Some women don't experience the typical night sweats, urinary frequency, hot flashes, and mood swings commonly seen. As a result, they develop a false sense of security believing everything to be perfectly fine. They actually are fortunate not to experience the symptoms associated with entering menopause, but the more serious effects are those not readily apparent.

Estrogens are very important for preventing demineralization of bone, as well as protecting the heart and blood vessels. The incidence of heart attacks increases dramatically after menopause. Without estrogen (estradiol in particular), the bones lose calcium and become more brittle and prone to fracture. That is the major reason why post-menopausal women sustain a much higher rate of fractures. It is not unusual to see patients who have sustained vertebral body compression fractures that result in the reduction in the height of the vertebrae. It is a very painful condition, but one that is *preventable*. It is also not unusual to learn that those females lose height as noted by comments like, "I used to be five foot five and I'm now five foot two." Multiple vertebral fractures can result in that very phenomenon. I remember the stories of menopausal women falling and fracturing their hips. The truth is, most fractured their hip and then fell. The bones fracture much more easily than normal because they have become so fragile with the loss of calcium. The developing condition is called osteopenia, and as it becomes more pronounced with additional calcium loss and boney demineralization; it's called osteoporosis.

Pharmaceutical companies have developed drugs to help prevent bone loss or to restore bone strength. There's certainly nothing wrong with marketing a product to maintain bone health, unless those drugs also have their own set of negative side effects. Women don't develop osteopenia and osteoporosis because of the lack of these drugs; it's because of the depletion of hormones. The most common drugs used to treat osteoporosis are Fosamax®, Actonel®, Boniva®, Reclast®, Atelvia®, and Evista®. All have side effects and some may cause muscle cramping, joint pain, atrial fibrillation (heart flutter), abdominal discomfort, and heart burn. One is tied to an increased incidence of pulmonary emboli (blood clots to the lung).

I return to the same question I have posed before by asking the obvious; if osteoporosis is not caused by the absence of the above listed drugs, then why take them? Why not treat the problem, instead, by supplementing with bioidentical hormones and reverse the problem by treating the cause? Remember, it was Prempro that was studied and reported in the Women's Health Initiative study, not bio-identical hormones! It is really very simple: women are menopausal because of the drop in estrogens, progesterone, and testosterone. In order to correct that deficiency and ward off the many ill effects associated with depleted hormones, **simply replace the hormones lost in the menopausal process!** Not only will it prevent bone loss and protect the heart, it will also maintain a number of other important functions and characteristics.

Most doctors understand that estrogen, particularly estradiol, is a hormone supplement to prescribe for menopausal or perimenopausal women. The reason why so much emphasis has been placed upon replacing estrogen only is the fact that many of the nuisance symptoms of menopause, such as night sweats and hot flashes, are due primarily to low estrogen, particularly estradiol. However, the hormones progesterone and testosterone are important as well.

I am always intrigued when female patients, who had undergone hysterectomies, tell me that their gynecologists neglected to prescribe either progesterone or testosterone. They were told they didn't need either because they no longer had a uterus. I find it intriguing, simply because it appears as though these gynecologists never learned about other organ systems. I assume it's because their teachers knew little about the subject either. Believe it or not, that is still being taught in obstetrics/gynecology residencies. Do they honestly believe that women have only one organ, the uterus? *Progesterone is important in women regardless of whether or not they have a uterus!* Progesterone tends to balance the system with estrogens. Menopausal women with low levels of progesterone can experience depression, insomnia, fatigue, joint pain, low sex drive, vaginal dryness, memory loss, and abdominal weight gain. Women who are still menstruating can experience all the above in addition to heavy menstruation and irregular cycles in the presence of low progesterone. In the menstruating female, progesterone's main function is to help ready the uterus for pregnancy by increasing the thickness of the endometrium, the inner lining of the uterus. Once the secretion of progesterone declines, the uterine lining is shed during a woman's period. Because of this single-minded focus, many gynecologists don't prescribe progesterone in women who have undergone a hysterectomy. The other factor is that estrogens have been linked to a higher incidence of uterine cancer, and if there's no uterus, then there's certainly no risk of uterine cancer.

Another questionable area is the many studies about chemicals/horse estrogens that people, including doctors, interpret to mean human hormones. It is confusing because terms are used interchangeably and reported in error. As an example, Prempro is not a bio-identical hormone; it contains horse estrogens and a chemical. Nevertheless, when reported in the news, the reference indicates that "hormones" were involved. There is no wonder why people are so confused. Regardless, **progesterone, not progestin, should always be used anytime a female takes estrogen to balance the system.**

Testosterone is also a very important hormone in the menopausal female, as well as in those females still menstruating. Testosterone is of utmost importance in the healing process. It is also very important if one wishes to achieve a positive response to exercise by increasing strength and endurance. It can assist in stabilizing the mood and preventing mood swings. It is similar to progesterone in assisting with mineralization of bone and preventing osteoporosis. The libido enhancing effects of testosterone are also present in the female, as well as the male. As an interesting illustration, it appears as though many doctors do not understand that the heart has more receptors for testosterone than any other organ system, with the exception of the reproductive system.

It is important to maintain all three sex hormones (estrogens, testosterone, and progesterone) at their optimum levels in order to achieve peak health with an optimum quality of life. As indicated above, the function of the estrogens, progesterone, and testosterone are many and are very important in combating the effects of aging. As always, it's an individual choice of how to spend later years of life. One can choose to be healthy and vibrant by supplementing lost hormones while adhering to proper eating habits and a regular exercise program. In contrast, one can also choose a lesser quality of life and complain of aches and pains, depression, mood swings, heart problems, bone mineral loss, loss of libido, and myriad other symptoms brought about as the result of declining hormones.

For females in their reproductive years, I see occasional problems brought about as the result of lower hormone levels, but it is infrequent. Everyone has heard the term PMS, (premenstrual syndrome). The hallmark of this syndrome is mood swings, but women may also have irregular periods or a heavy flow during their period. The problem can be treated by adding progesterone during the last part of their cycle, and stopped just before the anticipated menses. It is less common that estrogens or testosterone are too low in ovulating females, but it does happen.

Most female patients that require hormone replacement are perimenopausal or menopausal. Hormonal replacement for these ladies is entirely different from those who are ovulating regularly. Every prospective hormone replacement patient that comes to my office undergoes an initial consultation and discussion of various issues unique to them. They also undergo a number of serum (blood) tests to determine levels of pertinent hormones. In most cases, menopausal females have low levels of all sex hormones and commonly have suboptimal levels of free T3 (thyroid), manifested by low resting body temperatures. Critics of serum testing bring up the issue of it being only a "snapshot" in time for the hormone being tested. That is correct, because hormone levels vary throughout the day, but it allows us to check whether or not the level is within the optimal range.

When tested levels fall above or below the optimal range, it allows the doctor to determine whether or not to supplement that particular hormone. I have often been asked about saliva testing, but I have not found it to be as reliable as serum testing. Contrary to what proponents of saliva testing claim, the level of hormones seen in saliva do not necessarily reflect what is present in the blood and available at cellular receptor sites. It is the level seen in the blood that is of major importance, because that is how hormones are transported to receptor sites. For example, blood levels of progesterone may be reduced, while the level seen in the saliva is adequate or high. If a doctor were to accept the results of the saliva test alone, he/she might not prescribe progesterone in that patient, which would be a mistake. Because saliva testing has that margin of error when testing progesterone, I choose not to use it for testing any other hormones. A twenty-four hour urine collection actually offers the most accurate testing for hormone levels, but I do not use it for a number of reasons. I do not have a local laboratory that is able to provide results within a reasonable period of time. The specimen (urine) must be shipped out of state and then the results are typically delayed by two to three weeks. Not only is the test cumbersome, urine has to be collected for twenty-four hours; it is expensive as well. If the test was easily accessible, inexpensive, and had a shorter reporting time, I would use it exclusively. While serum testing is not perfect, it is also not cumbersome, is relatively inexpensive, and has a rapid turn-around time, but only provides a snapshot idea of hormone levels.

Once the serum levels are determined and then considered in conjunction with the patient's complaints and symptoms, I tailor a prescription regimen for each patient. The typical prescription is written for various doses of estradiol, progesterone, and testosterone. Usually all are combined in a cream or gel that is applied to the skin twice daily. The other methods include drops or lozenges that are absorbed through the mucosa of the mouth. It is not swallowed! It's important that the topical creams/gels are applied to areas of the body known to absorb to a greater extent. I routinely advise ladies to apply the creams/gels to the front of the neck, shoulders, and chest. The dosage regimen of the creams/gels, drops, or lozenges is twice a day everyday without breaks. Some doctors feel as though women should be given a break from hormones by simulating the menstrual cycle; however, I have not found that to be necessary in women who are no longer menstruating. I take into account the extra uterine benefits of each of the hormones, and have concluded that it is best to prescribe them to be used daily. Since the patient is no longer experiencing a menstrual cycle, mimicking something that does not exist is not necessary. Some may question why I do not also include the other two estrogens, estriol, and estrone, in the combination. Both are weaker estrogens, and the body will naturally convert some estradiol into estriol and estrone as needed. Accordingly, I rarely prescribe Biest or Triest, which simply describe whether or not the estrogen combination has two or three estrogens respectively.

The dosing schedule is somewhat different for the perimenopausal female who is still menstruating as opposed to those who have completed menopause. Estradiol is given in various dosages starting Day One of the cycle and continuing through Day Twenty twice daily. Day One is designated as the first day of the menstrual cycle. Starting on Day Fifteen, progesterone is given twice daily as well and that continues through Day Twenty-Five. Occasionally, I give progesterone once a day at bedtime if a patient complains of sleepiness after taking progesterone in the morning. Typically, the sleepiness becomes less of an issue with the passage of time. Testosterone is not cycled and is given twice a day, every day.

I typically do not use oral preparations of estrogens or testosterone, as it requires another step before being absorbed. Also, in the case of oral estrogens, it can result in an increased tendency for clotting, which can result in an increased incidence of strokes and heart attacks. When a hormone is taken by mouth, it must be absorbed through the gastrointestinal tract and then processed by the liver. However, when a hormone is absorbed through the oral mucosa or skin, the hormone is immediately available to the receptor site. I also do not use injections in females simply because it is typically unnecessary.

Pellets are another method of supplementing bioidentical hormones, but they are usually reserved for menopausal women who do not respond to other methods. Only estrogens and testosterone can be combined in a pellet, progesterone cannot. Dosages for pellets can't be reduced as opposed to dosages for creams or lozenges that can be changed very easily and quickly. Pellets release a certain amount of hormone gradually, and typically last about four to six months. If the laboratory results show too little of a particular hormone, then changing the dosage becomes a more challenging issue. For example, if a patient undergoes a procedure to place the rice grain-sized pellet under the skin and is subsequently found to have sub-optimal levels, then the dosage must be increased. The most viable way of accomplishing that is by the addition of a cream or lozenge. The pellet is typically implanted under the skin in the buttock. It requires numbing of the skin, allowing a painless small incision to be made, through which the pellet can be placed under the skin and closed with a Steri-strip. Pellets have the advantage of maintaining a more steady level of the hormone and the patient doesn't have to deal with replacement for 4-6 months. The other factor to consider about pellets is that progesterone cannot be included in a pellet and must be administered in another fashion. In other words, progesterone must be administered by using creams, capsules, drops, or lozenges. If the patient has to use a separate method of delivery for progesterone, then why not include everything at once? Why make it complicated? I realize that proponents of pellets, particularly gynecologists, advise women that progesterone is not necessary if they do not have a uterus, but this as noted previously, is simply not true. For patients whose gynecologist understands the importance of progesterone in women without a uterus, my advice is to continue under their care, provided they are willing to prescribe hormones that are identical to those made by the human body (bioidentical). Many gynecologists and other specialists have not investigated the evidence in favor of using bioidentical hormones. That doesn't make them bad people; it simply means they remain misinformed.

Critics of bioidentical hormone replacement therapy make the claim that bioidentical hormones have the same risk as their non-bioidentical counterparts. That claim is made in spite of having absolutely no evidence to support it.[4] If those groups are so concerned, why has a properly designed study in regard to bioidentical hormones not been performed? That would remove the doubt they have interjected and settle the debate. The reason, in my opinion, for not undertaking such a study is obvious. It's because the most probable outcome would be support for the use of bioidentical hormones as opposed to their non-bioidentical counterparts. As it is, the critics can continue to obscure the truth by continuing to speculate. The next time you hear a critic taking that stance, ask the simple question, why haven't the studies been done? The answer should be very interesting, but may not have a great deal to do with the actual truth. Are these critics front organizations, or silent supporters of the industry that has the most to gain from using patented replacements? That is a logical question, but I'm sure it would be difficult to get a valid answer. Debate can continue for years or decades, but for that debate to end properly, scientific evidence must be considered and applied logically. Critics of bioidentical hormones seem to be in favor of the status quo: pharmaceutical companies developing, manufacturing, and distributing all prescription preparations, including hormones or hormone look-alikes. Proponents of bioidentical hormones simply want a safe and viable alternative to non-bioidentical counterparts. Public records are available that provide undeniable evidence about numerous pharmaceutical companies purposely and knowingly allowing extremely dangerous drugs to be used by the vulnerable and unsuspecting public. Literally, **thousands** of innocent people have died or have been seriously injured as a result of this egregious behavior and blatant disregard for the lives of American citizens.[5] I have not heard of or read about anyone dying or sustaining any serious consequence as the result of taking bioidentical hormones. There is definitely something very wrong with the position taken by those who attempt to disparage bioidentical hormones as a safe and effective alternative. One only has to compare **thousands of deaths vs. no deaths!** In view of the tremendous disparity, this controversy seems to have developed as an attempt by the pharmaceutical industry (a.k.a. "Big Pharma"), to cast dispersions in order to divert attention from the real problem. This should be a simple exercise in the use of common sense, but the friends of Big Pharma don't intend to allow common sense to interfere with their self-serving stance. Some of Big Pharma's "friends" might surprise most people because many are representatives of well known organizations and government entities that make claims of putting patients first. It's always disappointing and surprising to discover what some people will do, or say, for money.

For patients who are still menstruating, I always check laboratory values of ferritin and B12. Ferritin is a protein complex that binds iron and either holds iron or releases it to be used in cellular functions. Iron is an essential component of hemoglobin that carries oxygen from the lungs to peripheral tissues. Since the menstrual period results in blood loss, it is simply logical to determine whether or not the blood loss has resulted in less than optimal levels of iron. Iron, B12, selenium, and zinc are also important factors in converting T4 to T3 (thyroid hormones). B12 also has a stabilizing effect on neuronal membranes (nerves) and is essential for proper DNA synthesis and fatty acid metabolism. Folic acid (B9) is another important vitamin that is used in conjunction with B12 and helps to control the accumulation of homocysteine, a reported risk factor for heart disease. Both B12 and folic acid can be ingested with a quality daily multiple vitamin compound, unless an absorption problem exists, such as in pernicious anemia. If an absorption problem exists, both B12 and folic acid can be injected on a weekly basis. For those females who have completed the climacteric (menopause) process and are no longer menstruating, the level of ferritin remains important, but is less of a concern, since it is no longer lost monthly.

My advice is to become proactive and ask questions about issues mentioned in this and other chapters. If you do not get the answers you know to be correct, then your alternative will be obvious. Find a doctor who actually has the answers, or is willing to become more educated. The only reason a doctor refuses to discuss bioidentical hormones is that he/she has no actual knowledge about this very important subject. Beware of a doctor who tells you that hormones are not necessary if you are not experiencing any symptoms beyond menopause as described in this chapter. If a doctor recommends starting estrogen supplementation, inquire as to whether or not he/she intends to prescribe progesterone and testosterone as well. The only exception to not prescribing progesterone and testosterone for all perimenopausal and menopausal females, is if the tested levels are truly adequate. That situation does occur, but it is uncommon. If he/she is willing to learn, you may consider remaining under their care, however, if they remain inflexible, it would be wise to immediately find another doctor. Any doctor who tells you that bioidentical hormones predispose you to cancer, heart disease, and stroke are not fully aware of the facts and have probably never taken the time to read and understand the actual studies. **No legitimate research study concerning a connection to cancer, stroke, or heart attack has ever been performed using bioidentical natural hormones.** Accordingly, it is simply speculation and opinion that natural bioidentical hormones cause any of those conditions. Be very careful whose opinion you rely upon, because much of that opinion can masquerade as being based upon science. In fact, many opinions are based upon pseudoscience, myths, speculation, and propaganda. Keep in mind that manufacturers of hormone look-alikes stand to lose revenue if patients begin using bioidentical hormones instead of their patented substitutes. Your doctor should know this, but it's what your doctor doesn't know that can hurt you.

Notes

[1] Kato, I. et al "Prospective study of factors influencing the onset of natural menopause." *Journal of Clinical Epidemiology*, 1998; 51:1271-1276.

[2] Vance D.A, "The Intriguing History of a Controversial Drug." *International Journal of Pharmaceutical Compounding*, 2007; 11(4):282-287.

[3] "Women's Health Initiative, Risks and benefits of estrogen plus progestin in healthy postmenopausal women." *Journal of the American Medical Association*, 2002; 288:321-333.

[4] Cirigliano, M. "Bioidentical hormone therapy: a review of the evidence." *Journal of Women's Health*, 2007;16(5):600-631.

[5] Evans, David, "When drug makers' profits outweigh penalties." *The Washington Post*, March 21, 2010; G01.

4

WHAT YOU NEED TO KNOW ABOUT HUMAN GROWTH HORMONE

There is a great deal of misinformation circulating about this particular hormone. As always, the misinformation can be traced to those who simply don't understand the facts, those who wish to remain in control by declaring themselves to be experts, or those who wish to profit at the expense of others. For many busy doctors, they simply believe what they are told or what they read, similar to most other people. If it's printed in a magazine, written in a book, or seen on television, then it must be true, right? Therein lies the problem for everyone; it's simply hard to separate fact from fiction. Accepted "authorities" spread incorrect information, while hucksters make claims that are simply false. The real truth lies somewhere in the middle of these contrasting camps.

Human growth hormone, or HGH, was unknown prior to the early 1900s. Even after doctors became aware that HGH existed, it took until the early 1950s to identify and isolate the actual HGH molecule from the human pituitary. By 1958, scientists had developed a method of extracting HGH from the pituitary glands of cadavers, which they then injected into children with stunted growth. The cadaver-derived HGH was successful in stimulating growth in those patients, and over 8,000 short statured children were treated from 1958 to 1985. Cadaver-derived HGH was discontinued in 1985 because of the report that several children had developed Creutzfeld-Jakob Disease from contaminated specimens. The disease results in deterioration of the central nervous system and is ultimately fatal. There was no screening method available to detect the virus causing the condition, resulting in doctors discontinuing the use of cadaver derived HGH. This led scientists to develop a method of synthesizing the same molecule through a very complicated DNA process and the end product was called recombinant DNA derived human growth hormone. All HGH used today is derived using this process, and as a result, no diseases can be passed on to anyone taking the preparation, as it is devoid of any infectious agents.[1]

A landmark study by Dr. Dan Rudman et al, was published in the *New England Journal of Medicine* in 1990 about the effects of recombinant DNA HGH on a small sample of men over the age of sixty, who were considered HGH deficient. The main point of the study was to determine whether or not there were positive effects of HGH in older men. The need in short stature children had already been established, but no study about the effects in older adults had ever been undertaken. Twelve healthy men between the ages of sixty and eighty-one were subjects of the study and received injections of HGH three times weekly for six months. There were also nine male subjects of similar age and health who received no treatment and functioned as the control group for the study. No changes were made in diet or exercise level in any of the subjects. The dosages of HGH were somewhat higher than what I typically use in HGH deficient patients, but the dosages did achieve those consistent with levels commonly noted in younger adult males. The reported results were rather striking, in that the men receiving HGH showed an average muscle mass gain of 8.8% and fat loss of 14.4%. A slight increase in bone density was also noted in the lumbar vertebrae (bones of the lower back) and a thickening of the skin was noted in the men receiving growth hormone. The study comments indicated, "These structural changes have been considered unavoidable results of aging. It has recently been proposed, however, that reduced availability of growth hormone in late adulthood may contribute to such changes." The study further summarized, "Diminished secretion of

HGH is responsible in part for decreased lean body mass, the expansion of adipose-tissue mass, and the thinning of the skin that occurs in old age."[2] The results of the study were overwhelmingly favorable and brought attention to the age-old concept and quest for the fountain of youth.

As noted earlier in this book, there is nothing that will reverse or stop the aging process, and those who make such claims about HGH are just as unscientific as those who claim it does nothing and should not be used in adults. It is an important hormone that is one piece of the puzzle in helping improve the quality of one's life.

On the one hand, there are the doctors who state that growth hormone should not be used in adults because of reasons that are based more upon personal bias, as opposed to actual science. There are members of that group who make claims that HGH causes cancer and diabetes. Those conditions have been mentioned in various studies, but no study has ever proven a definite connection. The claim that HGH causes cancer, or predisposes one to cancer, came about as the result of studies that showed patients who developed various forms of cancer, had also taken HGH in the past. For example, a study published in 1999 indicated that there was a higher level of IGF-1 found in lung, prostate, and breast cancers.[3] IGF-1 is a marker for the level of HGH and is typically reflective of the level of HGH in the system. It is secreted by the liver in response to the level of HGH. In other words, if the IGF-1 increases, it is because the level of HGH has also increased. Patients taking HGH show an increased level of IGF-1. Even though the study noted an increased level of IGF-1 in those particular cancers, it was concluded that, "While the studies indicate an association between serum IGF-1 levels and cancer risk, causality has not been established." Other studies have been performed as well, including one performed on patients who had been treated with cadaver derived HGH. Again, the study reported an increased incidence of colon and prostate cancer, but no definite connection to

IGF-1 or HGH was claimed.[4] It is important to note that particular study was a retrospective study on patients who had undergone treatment with *pituitary derived human growth hormone*. Creutzfeld-Jacob disease was passed on through contaminated pituitary derived HGH. For those who are genuinely scientifically inquisitive, the obvious question would be, what else was passed on through the contaminated specimens? Was an unidentified cancer producing agent passed on as well? I don't know the answer to that question, nor does anyone else. Not only have some opponents of HGH claimed that it causes cancer, but have jumped to the conclusion that prescribing HGH should be very restricted and prescribed only by qualified endocrinologists.[5] The stated goal of the Cancer Prevention Coalition is: "Our goal is to reduce escalating cancer rates through a comprehensive strategy of outreach, public education, advocacy, and public policy initiatives to establish prevention as the nation's foremost cancer policy." That is a worthwhile and commendable goal, provided it is sincere. The founder of the Coalition stated, "practitioners of this burgeoning 'health' (anti-aging medicine) industry are either ignorant of or suppress well-documented information on the grave cancer risks of HGH medication." Perhaps the founder is truly altruistic and concerned that HGH causes cancer, but it would seem that proof instead of hype would be the more scientific route to follow. I am also very curious why this same person has not sounded the alarm for women not taking iodine in sufficient doses? I question why iodine deficiency is not listed on the website of his Coalition. Is he ignorant or is he suppressing well-documented information on the grave risks of inadequate iodine intake? Surely he is not guilty of the same thing of which he accuses others! For more on that subject, refer to the chapter about hypothyroidism.

A few groups and individuals appear to be engaged in a crusade against the use of HGH in adults, for reasons unknown to me. Their views seem to be very slanted, as they magnify and focus on anything disparaging while minimizing the positive effects of HGH. Some of those groups are just as guilty of bias and misleading comments as are the hucksters and quacks who sell and promote anything to make a buck. We must all remain vigilant in regard to misstatements and hype because that takes place on both sides of the HGH issue with the truth lying somewhere between the two. Some of the "crusaders" claim to be non-profit organizations, so how do they pay their expenses? It appears as though one group advocates pharmacologic answers to virtually all ills and speaks against most natural remedies.[6] The same group does indeed expose fraudulent activities in the health care industry, but they are extremely one-sided and biased as they don't expose the ongoing fraud perpetrated by the pharmaceutical industry. The founder of that group vehemently denies receiving any funds from companies or individuals who might profit by his stance, and further minimizes the expenses necessary to continue his one-sided quest.

On the other side of the coin are the profit-motivated hucksters who have little or no concern about anyone's health. Since real HGH is relatively expensive, a new industry has evolved, supposedly for providing less expensive ways to increase levels of HGH. It is no wonder why so many people are confused about HGH! These same charlatans attempt to persuade the general public that they can effectively raise HGH levels by using substances that have HGH as an ingredient. They use slick advertising to promote their new "miracle" compounds that supposedly increase the level of HGH. Please note: the HGH molecule is far too large to be absorbed through the intestinal tract, the mouth, the nose, or the skin. Pills, tablets, nasal sprays, creams, or gels claiming HGH as an ingredient cannot and will not raise the level of HGH because it cannot be absorbed! The other fact to understand is that HGH is available only through a prescription. Accordingly, if there actually is any HGH in the preparation, it is an illegal substance without a prescription. The only way to administer HGH and actually raise the level of HGH is by injection. The question has been raised about how companies get away with such misleading advertising.

The answer lies in the manner in which their claims are worded. All of these companies talk about the positive effects of HGH and infer that their product will offer those results. The victims of the misleading commercial then order the product believing they will get the effects of increasing their level of HGH. If you listen carefully, you will find that the hucksters typically never indicate that the customer will increase their levels of HGH by taking their product, it was something the customer merely assumed. Listen to the words the next time you hear one of those commercials or read about such a product on the internet. Any company that makes a claim that their HGH containing product will raise your level of HGH is engaging in fraud.

Other products are referred to as secretagogues or substances that stimulate release of HGH from the pituitary. Most include the amino acids glutamine and arginine. Both amino acids have been shown to stimulate release of HGH from an intact functioning pituitary; however, they do little for a pituitary that is not producing enough HGH. Furthermore, the initial studies were performed using intravenous arginine, not oral. Some injectable secretagogues may stimulate release of HGH, but when the storage of HGH is exhausted and the pituitary lags behind in HGH production, then what? The answer is that the levels of HGH, regardless of stimulation, will fall to sub-optimal levels. There are also a few products that make the claim to not only stimulate the release of HGH, but to stimulate the production as well. I am not convinced that these products justify the claims, but would be open to reading and considering studies providing proof. There is no doubt that further research in this area is warranted.

I would estimate that over ninety percent of the websites about HGH on the internet are bogus and promote products that do not work. My advice is to exercise caution and engage in due diligence when considering the purchase of any product through the internet. For any patient who has documented adult growth hormone deficiency, I would advise using only prescribed injectable HGH. A secretagogue may achieve results for a short period of time, but injectable HGH is the only reliable way to truly increase blood levels.

Avoid any product that claims to have actual HGH as an ingredient because it is a scam. Injectable secretagogues typically work in a transient manner resulting in effects that are typically short-lived because they require a normal pituitary function. If a patient is truly growth hormone deficient, then that means the pituitary is not functioning at its peak efficiency and no secretagogue will correct that. In most cases, those who attempt to save money by shopping on the internet become victims of scammers.

Now that you understand what works, what doesn't work, and who is opposed to the use of HGH in adults by using scare tactics to make their point, it's time to understand the truth and facts about HGH. Human growth hormone is not a miracle drug, nor will it reverse or stop the aging process! It is simply a 191 amino acid chain hormone that is secreted naturally by every normal person's pituitary gland. It is the hormone that determines one's height, but continues to remain useful even when one reaches their ultimate height. The problem is that it is secreted on a less gradual basis as one ages. Because of its declining presence, the positive effects also decline at the same rate. Again, it is not a miracle hormone, but it has a number of positive effects. The initial studies on adults showed that HGH resulted in increased muscle mass, reduced fat tissue, and increased bone density when administered to men over the age of sixty who were treated for six months.[7] Perhaps even more important is the fact that studies have revealed that HGH results in an improvement of immune function.[8] Earlier studies showed that HGH resulted in reversing shrinkage of the thymus gland which is an extremely important gland for immune function.[9] The thymus gland shrinks gradually throughout life, but no one understood exactly why. Now we believe that the shrinkage is directly related to one's level of circulating HGH.

Other studies have reached the same conclusion in regard to HGH and its immune-enhancing effects. HGH has been shown to stimulate the cellular proliferation of lymphoid organs (bone marrow, thymus) and activate peripheral lymphocytes and macrophages.

HGH was studied in regard to its role in healing after surgery and enhancement of the immune system as well.[10] The study showed HGH to extend the life of white blood cells known as PMNs (poly-morphonuclear neutrophils) that play a very important positive role in promoting healing. The prolonged life of those cells also resulted in an improvement of immune function.

HGH administration also improves heart function.[11] Deficiency of HGH was associated with a significantly greater degree of dysfunction in cardiac output as compared to those with higher levels of HGH. Only twenty-one percent of those with HGH deficiency showed normal cardiac function, as compared to 93% in those with no deficiency. Not only did the cardiac function improve with HGH supplementation, but the risk factors for heart disease also improved. Both lipoprotein (a) and C-reactive protein were noted to decrease in those treated with HGH.[12] It was also observed that those with HGH deficiency were significantly more prone to develop atherosclerotic vascular disease (hardening of the arteries). Opponents of HGH often make claims that administration of recombinant DNA HGH can cause diabetes. In fact, research has shown the opposite as HGH tends to reduce the incidence of adult onset diabetes mellitus by reducing insulin resistance.[13]

Other than laboratory testing, how does one recognize whether or not they have human growth hormone deficiency? Many symptoms and signs of adult HGH deficiency overlap with those caused by sub-optimal function of other endocrine organs and can be quite confusing. However, as one ages, the probability of developing adult HGH deficiency increases because pituitary output of HGH diminishes about fourteen percent per decade once puberty is finished. The following are a number of signs and symptoms that may result from declining levels of HGH. The physical examination typically reveals evidence of thinning fragile skin with wrinkling (most notably in the back of the hands), an increased percentage of body fat, and a reduction in muscle mass. Much of the fat gain is around the middle, referred to as central adiposity. Since HGH has a positive effect on the immune system, as noted above, those with HGH deficiency may begin to notice more frequent colds or unexplained low grade illnesses with or without fever. Those with HGH deficiency frequently complain of sleep problems as well. Many patients are able to sleep, but state that they don't seem to be able to get restful sleep.[14] Demineralization of bone (osteopenia or osteoporosis) can also become worse with HGH deficiency. Those conditions are typically seen in older female patients who are much more prone to sustaining needless painful fractures. The most common fractures occur in the spine (vertebral bodies), but fractures also occur in other areas as well. Older males are subject to this risk as well, but it is less common.

Patients who seek to undergo treatment for adult growth hormone deficiency should first be evaluated properly by a qualified physician. The history is a very important part of that evaluation. A history includes many things, but allows the doctor to become more familiar with one's complaints, symptoms, medical history, medications being taken, family history, allergies, work history, level of education, and other things that might be overlooked with a physical examination only. Next would be a physical examination assessing all body systems. Once the physical examination is completed, appropriate laboratory testing should be performed. If the patient's history, physical examination, and laboratory studies indicate adult growth hormone deficiency, the doctor may then prescribe synthesized recombinant HGH for the patient. I typically prescribe two to three micrograms per kilogram of body weight for each patient to inject daily. One microgram (mcg) is 1,000,000th of one gram as opposed to a milligram that is 1,000th of one gram. If a person weighs 200 pounds that means they weigh ninety-one kilograms (kg). Multiply ninety-one by two and the answer is 182 mcgs or .182 mg. Confused yet? Multiply ninety-one by three and the answer is 273 mcg or .273mg. Those are the daily doses for a person weighing 200 pounds. For those who are growth hormone deficient, I typically start their dosage at .2mg daily. The HGH is injected subcutaneously (under the skin) using a very small needle. Instructions are given on how to inject daily, and even the most squeamish seem to adapt very easily. Because of the relatively small dosage, there is no reason to skip days. Some physicians advise injecting five days and taking two days off, but it is really not necessary as the only thing accomplished would be to deprive the patient of HGH for two days.

The patient is then re-evaluated six to eight weeks later and the level of HGH is again determined. The doctor will then be able to assess whether or not the dosage is appropriate and may increase the dosage if indicated. I have rarely found it necessary to increase the dosage beyond 0.6mg per day, with most patients remaining at the 0.2 to 0.4mg dosage level per day. The only exception has been grossly obese patients or those patients of large stature.

Patients are also monitored for nuisance side effects such as peripheral edema (swelling of the hands or feet) or a skin reaction at the injection site. For those patients who have underlying carpal tunnel syndrome, it is not unusual for them to experience an exacerbation (worsening) of their symptoms if they are in the group of patients that have swelling. Carpal tunnel syndrome is a condition in which the median nerve is pinched in the wrist causing tingling, numbness, and/or pain in the thumb, forefinger, and middle finger of the hand. Swelling can make those symptoms worse because it can reduce the size of the canal through which the nerve passes. In opposition to what some authorities claim, HGH does not cause carpal tunnel syndrome, but it can definitely make an existing condition worse. If one experiences a skin reaction at the injection site, they are advised to stop the injections for a week and then resume. The incidence of swelling (water retention) is very low, but if it occurs, the patient is instructed to not use HGH injections for one week and resume using a lesser dosage beginning the second week and remain on that dose for two weeks. After that, the patient may resume the normal dosage unless the side effect symptoms return. It is rare, but some patients simply can't tolerate the side effects of HGH, even though they may be growth hormone deficient.

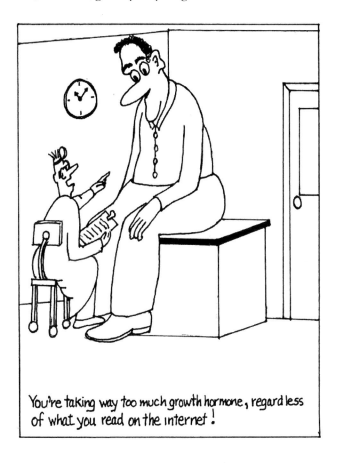

You're taking way too much growth hormone, regardless of what you read on the internet!

A condition known as acromegaly exists and it results from excessive HGH. Typically, the condition is the result of an HGH secreting pituitary adenoma (tumor), but it can also occur if a person injects excessive HGH over a period of months.

When youngsters complete puberty, the long bones fuse and additional linear growth cannot occur. A person's height is determined by that time and administering HGH after that time will not result in any additional increase in height. When there is too much HGH after the time the long bones have fused, the only direction the bones can grow is in width. With acromegaly, the bones of the forehead, knuckles, wrists, and lower jaw grow in width. There is also associated soft tissue swelling and thickening of the skin, with noticeable enlargement of the hands, feet, lips, ears, and nose. Soft tissue swelling also occurs internally as well and can affect the internal organs. Many victims of this disease suffer from enlargement of the heart with associated congestive heart failure. It can also affect the vocal cords resulting in a deepening of the voice. Acromegaly will not occur as the result of treatment with the low treatment doses previously mentioned for those that are growth hormone deficient.

I believe that Sergeant Joe Friday, of Dragnet fame, said it best, "Just the facts ma'am, just the facts." When the smoke has cleared, I believe HGH will take its place beside other hormones that help maintain a higher quality of life for aging individuals. The controversy has arisen because biased people use pseudoscience to back their claims on both sides of the issue of whether or not to use HGH in adults. HGH is a hormone secreted by the pituitary of all human beings. It normally declines with age until the symptoms of low growth hormone levels begin to appear. When that occurs, it is a hormone that can be supplemented in order to help alleviate the symptoms previously noted in this chapter. When HGH is used in a judicious and prudent manner in patients who are growth hormone deficient it is simply another piece of the puzzle that will help improve their health and quality of life. When a person is involved in a complete healthy living program with optimization of all hormones, adherence to a proper way of eating, and includes a regular exercise program, it follows that the person will look better, feel better, and be less likely to succumb to the many ills suffered by those who don't follow such a program. In a healthy aging program, it has often been said that HGH is the icing on the cake as it overlaps and assists with the action of other hormones. It is logical to assume that a person that is more healthy will live longer, but the jury is still out on that particular subject. Regardless, there will always be the hucksters and con artists making claims that are not supported by science on one end of the spectrum while the self-proclaimed experts warn against all the negative possible side effects on the other end. Somewhere in the middle the truth resides, and remember, what your doctor doesn't know can hurt you.

Notes

[1] Gardner, D. et al, *Greenspan's Basic and Clinical Endocrinology*, (8th edition) 2007: New York-McGraw-Hill Medical: pp 193-201.

[2] Rudman, D. et al "Effects of Human Growth Hormone in Men Over 60 Years Old." *New England Journal of Medicine*, July 1990; 323(1):1-6

[3] Shim, M. and Cohen, P. "IGFs and human cancer, implications regarding the risk of growth hormone therapy." *Hormone Research.*, 1999; 51(3):42-51.

[4] Swerdlow, AJ et al, "Risk of cancer in patients treated with human pituitary growth hormone in the UK, 1959-1985: a cohort study." *Lancet*, July 2002; 360(9329): 273-277.

[5] Epstein S., "Human Growth Hormone (hGH) medications increase risks of colon, prostate and breast cancer." Cancer Prevention Coalition. Website March 2000.

[6] Barrett, Steven, Quackwatch.org.

[7] Rudman, D. et al "Effects of Human Growth Hormone in Men Over 60 Years Old." *New England Journal of Medicine*, July 1990; 323(1):1-6

[8] Gelato M.C., "Growth Hormone-Insulin Growth Factor I and Immune Function." *Trends Endocrinol. Metab*, April 1993; 4(3):106-110.

[9] Kelley K.W. et al "GH3 pituitary adenoma can reverse thymic aging in rats." *Proceedings of the National Academy of Science USA*, Aug 1986;83(15):5663-5667.

[10] Decker, D. et al "Perioperative treatment with human growth hormone down-regulates apoptosis and increases superoxide production in the PMN from patients undergoing infrarenal abdominal aortic aneurysm repair." *Growth Hormone IGF Research*, June 2005; (15):193-199.

[11] Gola, M. et al "Growth Hormone and Cardiovascular Risk Factors." *Journal of Endocrinology and Metabolism*, Dec 2004; 90(3):1864-1870.

[12] Sesmilo, G. et al "Effects of GH administration in inflammatory and other cardiovascular risk markers in men with GH deficiency." *Annals of Internal Medicine*, July 2000; 133(2):111-122.

[13] Christian, J. "Effects of GH upon Body Composition." *Growth Hormone in Adults*, 1996; Cambridge University Press.

[14] Van Cauter, E. et al "Interrelationships Between Growth Hormone and Sleep." *Growth Hormone IGF Research*, April 2000; Suppl B:557-562.

5

ROLE OF THE ADRENAL GLANDS

We use the term "stress," in regard to our health, to describe a situation in which pressure, tension, or strain is brought to bear upon us and how it affects us emotionally and physically. Stress occurs for many reasons, not the least of which is the pressure involved with the activities of everyday life. It would take an entire book to describe the many causes of stress (stressors). For example, ask yourself if you have ever been sad because of the loss of a friend, family member, or colleague. That sadness is normal, but it also is stressful. A negative change in a friendship, a relationship, or an occupation can result in various degrees of stress for the individual involved. Every person deals with emotional stress in their own way. The same holds true for physical stress such as when one is sick or injured. Those situations are very stressful for the person involved, but it is also stressful for those related to or associated with that person. Environment stressors, such as pollution and toxins, can also stimulate a similar response physiologically. Stress provoking situations are around us all and it is going to continue. I've heard many people say, "I wish I could move and get away from all this stress." Ironically, upon moving, other stressors appear that result in a similar emotional and physiological response. In other words, it is a part of living and it is each person's prerogative to deal with it effectively or allow it to rule their life.

Obviously, one should avoid stressors when possible, but regardless of dedicated efforts, stress will still be a part of life. With that in mind, one should implement ways to deal with or reduce stress. It is wise to recognize that life will never be stress free, so one should not allow stressful situations to become more stressful by assuming a victim attitude. Just accept stress as a part of life and that alone will help in reducing your body's response to stress. One can reduce stress by setting aside times to relax using whatever technique works best for them. A variety of relaxation methods are listed in books, magazines, websites etc. A regular exercise program, such as walking, yoga, or swimming, is a tried and true method of stress reduction. However, engaging in excessive exercise activities can induce stress. Others choose to read, meditate, play a musical instrument, utilize visualization techniques, etc. The list goes on and on for activities designed to accomplish the end result of stress reduction through relaxation or diversion of attention.

Eating properly is of utmost importance as well. The proper way to eat is described in the chapter, "Your Are What You Eat." One can't expect to be free of stress and eat incorrectly. Incorrect eating habits will increase stress simply by maintaining a relatively unbalanced eicosanoid (short-acting hormone) system. When discussing diet, it is interesting and ironic to me that most people who make the claim that they eat properly are most guilty of engaging in the worst eating habits. People believe marketing and forget the basic concept of proper eating as the result of proper macronutrient balance. If the package says, "fortified with all essential vitamins and minerals," most believe the product to be healthy. Another term that confuses many people is "organic." Simply because a food product says fortified or organic has no bearing on whether or not the food is healthy, particularly in regard to macronutrient balance. Organic is a term used to designate that a product is essentially free from unwanted chemicals including fertilizers and pesticides. It is healthier than consuming products having the potential of containing chemicals, but it doesn't guarantee a proper short-acting hormone response to that food. When the proper balance of macronutrients (protein, fat, and carbohydrate) are maintained, that results in better health and reduces stress.

Organic foods are superior to their counterparts, but the macronutrient balance is the key. When balance is achieved, the additional stressor of an improper diet is reduced or avoided.

Rest is also very important in regard to dealing with stress. Without proper rest, stressors tend to evoke a greater physiological response within that person. We've all heard the term, "burning the candle at both ends." That term was coined for those people who were not dealing with stress appropriately. Typically, stress rules the life of people who personify that term. They typically do not eat right, don't avoid stress, don't attempt to reduce stress, and they don't get proper rest. They are simply a disaster waiting to happen.

Another area of stress reduction has to do with many of the chapters in this book about hormonal replacement. Optimal hormonal balancing is an absolutely necessary component of dealing with stress. The stress of inadequate hormones in the system is certainly not healthy for the reasons listed in each chapter, but suboptimal hormone levels also result in stress. When hormones are not optimal, the body functions that are directly related to those particular hormones are impaired. When impairment of any normal body function exists, it will result in stress provocation that can ultimately lead to the development of adrenal fatigue.

The question remains, what actually happens to the body when stress is allowed to continue unabated? Physiologic response is a term that designates what happens to the body when stress is not reduced or dealt with in a proper manner. A few examples of a physiologic response are things such as increased sweating, hyperventilation, changes in blood pressure, changes in pulse rate, trembling, anxiety, fear, etc. When I see a patient who is experiencing unexplained and inappropriate physiological responses such as those noted, adrenal fatigue is certainly something to be considered. I discuss stress avoidance or reduction, diet, regular low level exercise, and proper rest. Once a patient implements those needed changes, improvement sometimes takes place. I also implement appropriate hormonal optimization when indicated. However, some patients still feel "wired and tired," in spite of making needed changes and those are the ones who require additional assistance because the stress may have resulted in adrenal fatigue. Adrenal fatigue is a term that is based upon the body's inability to "keep up" with the many stressors in some patient's lives, resulting in the inability to secrete hormones necessary for optimal health.

The adrenal glands are small, triangular-shaped endocrine organs that sit atop the kidneys. The gland itself is composed of a cortex (covering) and a medulla (inner core). The function of the cortex is to secrete aldosterone (maintains proper blood pressure), cortisol, and dihydroepiandrosterone (DHEA), with small amounts of estradiol and testosterone. The adrenal medulla secretes epinephrine and norepinephrine. For the patients in whom I suspect adrenal fatigue, I test serum levels of total cortisol (preferably in the morning) and DHEA because aldosterone deficiency is typically not an issue. If the lab values for cortisol and DHEA are less than optimal, I then institute a program of replacement. In some cases, I will perform an adrenal challenge test in order to determine the ability of the adrenal cortex to secrete cortisol. Aldosterone deficiency is suspected when the patient's blood pressure remains very low after supplementing with cortisol and DHEA. When present, it can be treated with fludrocortisone that is known by the brand name, Florinef®. The causes of aldosterone deficiency are many and are not necessarily the result of adrenal fatigue.[1]

There are numerous symptoms suggestive of adrenal fatigue, but most people describe symptoms that fall within the "wired and tired" category. The patients appear anxious and many complain of anxiety, but have no energy. They typically have difficulty getting restful sleep and often state it's because the "wheels keep turning," even when attempting to sleep. They go to bed tired and wake up tired. As a result, it becomes a vicious cycle that must be broken. It is also not unusual to see low blood pressure in suspected adrenal fatigue patients that may return to normal levels with supplementation of cortisol and DHEA. Adrenal fatigue can mask an underlying hypothyroidism, but the adrenal fatigue component must be treated before addressing the thyroid issue.

In patients who have suspected adrenal fatigue with associated cortisol deficiency, I typically prescribe physiological doses of hydrocortisone (a.k.a. cortisol). It is important for patients and doctors alike to understand the term "physiological" and how it differs from "pharmacological." The adrenals secrete between eight to twenty-eight mg of cortisol daily, depending upon the source one reads.[2][3] Physiological doses simply refer to supplementation with low dose cortisol in an attempt to mimic normal levels. Pharmacological refers to supplementing with doses of cortisol-like substances that exceed normal levels of adrenal secretion. Cortisol is normally secreted by the adrenal cortex in small bursts, and it is known that morning levels of cortisol are generally higher than at any other time. As a result, I advise patients to take their hydrocortisone in the morning upon rising. Since cortisol does not stay very long in the system (half-life), they are usually dosed again in the early afternoon. One must take into account that not all hydrocortisone taken will be absorbed. Patients taking 2.5 to 5mg does not mean they will absorb that amount into their system. The typical dosing schedule is 1.25 to 2.5mg twice daily as noted. It is difficult to determine the exact amount required by each patient simply because there are variables that make each patient unique. Dosages are typically determined based upon the response of the patient.

The obvious question that begs an answer is why do we need cortisol and why is it important to know when it is low? Cortisol assists in maintaining proper levels of blood sugar by assisting in the breakdown of glycogen (stored glucose) in the liver, but it also inhibits glucose utilization peripherally (insulin resistance).[4] In turn, glucose is the fuel that drives the engine (cellular mechanism), allowing the continuation of all body processes. Cortisol also prevents sodium loss through the small intestine of mammals. The maintenance of proper levels of sodium assists in maintaining proper pH balance. However, sodium loss does not affect cortisol levels. Excess cortisol can result in retention of sodium that can result in increased blood pressure and it can also increase vascular response to epinephrine and norepinephrine. In essence, normal cortisol levels help to maintain normal blood pressure. Cortisol can also cause diuresis (loss of water) through the small intestine.[5] Excess cortisol can result in the impairment of calcium absorption in the small intestine and may lead to reduced bone formation with the development of osteoporosis.[6]

Excess cortisol can also inhibit the immune system by interfering with the formation of T- cells, but has no effect on natural killer cells.[7] [8] It also assists in the well-known process of reducing inflammation by reducing histamine secretion and the tendency for cells to rupture and release inflammatory components into the tissue.

There are a number of factors that may result in increased cortisol production, such as sleep deprivation, severe trauma or illness, anorexia nervosa, excessive caffeine, excess estrogen or melatonin in post-menopausal women, subcutaneous fat storage, and any stressful activity of daily living such as commuting, having to tolerate heavy traffic, domestic conflict, etc. Increased cortisol is not a problem if it is temporary. The problem arises when cortisol remains elevated secondary to any cause. In most cases, cortisol elevation can be reversed with dancing, laughing, crying, taking magnesium, fish oil, vitamin C, listening to certain types of music, and sexual intercourse, just to mention a few.

DHEA is a steroid hormone that has reported effects of improving memory, clarity of thinking, and mood.[9] Because of its conversion into the metabolite testosterone, DHEA may also help to restore muscle mass and strength, as well as providing a protective effect against (atherosclerosis) hardening of the arteries.[10] DHEA is also an important hormone for enhancing fertility in women.[11] It has also been observed to possibly promote the life span of those taking supplemental DHEA.[12]

To summarize, adrenal fatigue, as indicated, is characterized primarily by decreased levels of cortisol and DHEA because of the reported inability of the adrenal glands to "keep up" with adequate secretion. Engaging in activities mentioned during the first part of this chapter will assist the patient in reducing stress to the extent of not over taxing the adrenal glands. However, in many cases, the patient will need to be placed on hydrocortisone and DHEA supplementation in addition to exercising, learning stress avoidance or reduction and following a proper diet.

Notes

[1] Arai, K. et al, "Aldosterone Deficiency and Resistance-Chapter 24," www.endotext.org., April 28, 2010.

[2] Estaban, E.V. et al. "Daily cortisol production rate in man determined by stable isotope dilution/mass spectrometry," *J Clin Endocrinol Metab.* 1991 Jan;72(1):39-45.

[3] Miloro, G.E. et al., *Peterson's principles of oral and maxillofacial surgery.* Volume 1, 2004;B.C. Decker, Inc., Hamilton,Ontario.

[4] United States Medical Licensing Examination (USMLE) Step1 Secrets 2003. p. 63.

[5] Sandle, G.I. et al, "The effect of hydrocortisone on the transport of water, sodium and glucose in the jejunum. Perfusion studies in normal subjects and patients with coeliac disease." *Scand J. Gastroenterol.* 16(5):667-671.

[6] Shultz, T.D. et al, "Decreased calcium absorption in vivo and normal brush membrane vesicle calcium uptake in cortisol-treated chickens: evidence for dissociation of calcium absorption from brush border vesicle uptake," *Proc. Natl. Acad. Sci. U.S.A.,* 79(11):3542-3546.

[7] Palacios, R. et al "Hydrocortisone abrogates proliferation of T-cells in autologous mixed lymphocyte reaction by rendering the interleukin-2 Producer T-cells unresponsive to interleukin and unable to synthesize the T-cell growth factor." *Scand. J. Immunol.* 1982; 15(1):25-31.

[8] Onsrud, M. et al, "Influence of in vivo hydrocortisone on some human lymphocyte subpopulations. I. Effect on natural killer cell activity." *Scand. J. Immunol.* 1981; 13(6):573-579.

[9] Young, E.A. et al, "Increased evening activation of the hypothalamic-pituitary-adrenal axis in depressed patients." *Archives of General Psychiatry.* 1994; 51(9):701-707.

[10] Fukui, M. et al, "Serum dehydroepiandrosterone sulfate concentration and carotid atherosclerosis in men with type 2 diabetes." *Atherosclerosis,* 2005; 181(2):339-344.

[11] Casson, P.R. et al, "Dehydroepiandrosterone supplementation augments ovarian stimulation in poor responders: a case series." *Hum Reprod.* 2000;15: 2129-2132.

[12] Enomoto, Mika et al, "Serum Dehydroepiandrosterone sulfate Levels Predict Longevity in Men: 27-Year Follow-Up Study in a Community Based Cohort. (Tanushimaru Study)" *Journal of the American Geriatrics Society,* 2008; 56(6):994-998.

6

YOU ARE WHAT YOU EAT

There is no mystery why so many people are confused about how and what to eat. The information available is conflicting in spite of being generated by so-called authorities in the field of nutrition. Many highly credentialed authors cite research evidence to support their claims, but if one takes the time to check, they may find little credibility with what is claimed. It's very easy to influence uninformed people simply by stating, "Studies have shown…" What studies? Was there really a study, and if so, was it properly designed and performed? One of the most popular low fat "diet gurus" has published several books and is frequently a guest on radio and T.V. shows about nutrition. The only problem is that this "diet guru" is dead wrong in recommending a low fat diet. There are only three macronutrients, protein, fat, and carbohydrates (carbs). It is the ratio of these macronutrients that is so vitally important in regard to your health.

The rumor and movement pushing the low fat diet craze began in 1953 with an article in the *Journal of Mount Sinai Hospital* entitled "Atherosclerosis: a problem in newer public health" written by Ancel Keys, PhD. He observed that plaque within artery walls was composed of cholesterol and calcium. Unfortunately, he reported that eating saturated fat resulted in high levels of cholesterol that led to heart disease through the development of atherosclerosis, or what's commonly known as hardening of the arteries. I say unfortunately, because his conclusion was wrong then and studies have finally proven it to be wrong again and again. His study was very poorly designed. He seemed to have had a foregone conclusion that high fat diets resulted in increased blood cholesterol that caused heart disease. He sought out countries that had high intakes of fat and a high incidence of heart disease. He originally found twenty-two countries that consumed high percentages of fat, but he reported only six that had a high incidence of heart disease because they were the only ones to fit his theory. Instead of reporting the facts as he found them, he chose to ignore the remaining sixteen countries, even though they had a population that consumed a high percentage of fat in their diets, but had a lower incidence of coronary heart disease! That information was the basis of recommending a low fat diet for President Eisenhower after he had a heart attack. His cholesterol level at the time of his first heart attack was 151 and that is well within normal limits by today's standards. Regardless, the low fat craze overcame commonsense, the President's cholesterol level increased, and of course, most people know that he finally succumbed to a fatal heart attack. That wasn't enough for Dr. Keys. Not only did he get his fraudulent "Six Country" article published, but he repeated the same scientific dishonesty in 1970 when he published his so-called "Seven Countries Study." In that study, again Dr. Keys just ignored countries that didn't support his conclusion. He looked at fifteen countries, but found only seven that actually supported his theory. Regardless, he submitted his "Seven Countries Study" for publication even though he knew the design was unscientific. Those two articles led to years of misinformation and misunderstanding about the true cause of heart disease and hardening of the arteries. The theory, unscientific as it has been proven to be, was taught to new doctors in training and is still accepted as fact among doctors even though the questionable nature of the study design has been exposed and the theory challenged. Many physicians still contend that diets, high in saturated fat and cholesterol, cause heart disease. In 1991, statistician Russell H. Smith published a report entitled "Diet, Blood Cholesterol, and Coronary Heart Disease" in which he discussed the "Seven Countries Study." He stated,

"The dietary assessment methodology was highly inconsistent across cohorts and thoroughly suspect. In addition, careful examination of the death rates and associations between diet and death rates reveal a massive set of inconsistencies and contradictions… **It is almost inconceivable that the Seven Countries study was performed with such scientific abandon.** It is also dumbfounding how the NHLBI/AHA (National Heart, Lung and Blood Institute/American Heart Association) alliance ignored such sloppiness in their many "rave reviews" of the study… In summary, the diet-CHD relationship reported for the Seven Countries study cannot be taken seriously by the objective and critical scientist."[1]

Accordingly, saturated fat and cholesterol are NOT killing people! That is like saying that cars cause car accidents and are killing people. Cholesterol is not the villain that it has been portrayed to be. It does not cause plaque formation; it simply becomes a component of the plaque and then gets the blame. Most physicians become extremely excited if a patient's cholesterol level is reported over 200. The reason is because they continue to believe the old myth that has never been proven. This same myth is being perpetuated by the pharmaceutical industry that makes billions of dollars selling potentially toxic cholesterol-lowering agents that you hear about every day and night on television. Why doesn't your doctor know the truth? Most don't know any better because they received incorrect information during their years of training and afterwards as well. There are still doctors writing, in my opinion, misleading books about the hazards of higher cholesterol that advocate low fat diets in order to correct the problem. More specifically, many recommend reducing the intake of cholesterol and saturated fat while saying nothing about trans-fats like margarine and vegetable oils. Unfortunately, the very people who should know better, the cardiologists (heart doctors), are some of the greatest proponents of this myth.

In all but the most egregious circumstances, I think it is unprofessional and rude to mention other physicians' names in a disparaging way, but there are a few diet "gurus" that have, in my opinion, continued to spread incorrect and dangerous information that a low fat diet is the best and most healthy diet. Nothing could be further from the truth because saturated animal fat and cholesterol, does not cause heart disease! To the contrary, some fat is necessary for good health and the antiquated idea that dietary fat clogs the arteries is absolute nonsense not supported by scientific fact. Regardless of the truth, these self-appointed experts continue their arrogant quest of spreading rumors to the ill-informed. With people like that gaining prominence, is it any wonder why many people remain confused? Some of these same experts are gradually changing their hard stance toward eating fat. After a few years, these same people will try to convince the public who buy their books that it was them who finally discovered that a low fat or no fat diet was unhealthy. These types are simply opportunists, and if you truly want to know who they are, just go to your local bookstore and look for the books that advocate low fat diets. You may be very surprised when you discover who they are because it's the same bunch that seem to show up on all the TV shows since they're the ones we all know as the "experts." That's a pretty scary situation. The low fat "experts" have been giving out dangerous information for years, but they are still considered experts. So, if you really choose to increase your chances of living a shorter life, go get one of their books and follow it verbatim. Remember, it's what your doctor doesn't know that can hurt you!

If fat is not the villain it has been portrayed to be, then what has been causing health problems for many of us? For this particular subject, a lot has been learned from ancient man. Studies of ancient mummified remains by paleopathologists have shown little evidence of cancer, heart disease, or stroke. Mummies are much more plentiful than most people realize since most believe that it was only the Egyptians who preserved the remains of the deceased. Cultures had been mummifying the remains of the deceased for thousands of years before Egyptian civilization became so prominent on the world scene. It was the study of the non-Egyptian remains that shed a great deal of light on the importance of diet in regard to health and helped destroy the myth that low fat diets were the best and most healthy way of eating. Contrary to popular opinion, obesity was quite prevalent in Egyptian society and the first written account of a heart attack was discovered in Egyptian literature. It is also known that Egypt was one of the world's first agrarian (farming) societies as opposed to previous societies that were primarily of the "hunter-gatherer" variety. One of Egypt's primary food staples was grain from which bread was produced.[2] As the result of eating excessive amounts of bread, hence high glycemic carbohydrates (carbs), Egyptian citizens consistently raised their insulin levels to much higher levels than had ancient man.

It is the consistently high insulin levels that contributed to the development of many diseases such as heart disease, cancer, and stroke. High insulin levels are not dangerous unless they remain elevated on a consistent and prolonged basis. Many maintain consistently elevated insulin levels by consuming only carbohydrates or a diet with a high percentage of carbs; as one should begin to understand, this is not the best thing to do for one's health. Regardless, the first high carb diet was born in Egypt and people began to die prematurely as a result and obesity became the rule rather than the exception. One would think that modern day man would learn lessons from history, but because of ignorance, arrogance, and profit, it seems as though we must learn the same lessons again. Over the last two to three decades, our society has seen an explosion in obesity with more and more people getting fatter and fatter and the incidence of type II diabetes exploding. Take a walk down a city street just to see for yourself.

You may ask yourself why insulin, that is otherwise necessary for life, is such a problem. Insulin is made and secreted by the pancreas which is an organ located in the upper abdominal cavity. Insulin is necessary to help transport glucose into cells to be used as an energy source. The creation of energy that can be used by your body, involves a complex chemical reaction (Krebs cycle) once the glucose reaches the mitochondria of the cell. If there is not enough insulin, then glucose will remain in the blood and the cells will be deprived of their energy source. On the other hand, what if there is too much insulin? Excessive insulin will reduce the level of glucose in the blood to lower levels and the individual becomes hypoglycemic (insufficient glucose in the blood). Symptoms of hypoglycemia include fatigue, difficulty concentrating, sleepiness, memory issues, lethargy, and a craving for carbs. That is why many people experience afternoon "sinking spells" requiring some to take quick naps. When insulin spikes as the result of eating all carbs or too high a ratio of carbs, it results in the so-called "yo-yo effect," whereby the glucose is high then low and high again when the person consumes carbs to combat the feeling of fatigue normally associated with this condition. Too much insulin also interferes with the body's production of short acting hormones known as eicosanoids and an unbalanced system can wreak havoc upon one's health. Eicosanoids were not discovered until the mid-1980s, so it would not be unusual if you have not heard this term. Insulin is also a **fat storage hormone** and the longer insulin stays elevated, the harder it is for a person to lose weight, pure and simple!

Now that you know that you raise your insulin levels by eating carbs, what is the best way to lower your insulin requirement and insulin level? The obvious answer is to reduce your intake of carbs. However, all carbs are not the same in regard to the way they affect your need for insulin. Some carbs enter your bloodstream very quickly while others are much slower. This concept is referred to as the glycemic index, and just to make it simple, let's refer to carbohydrates as fast if they enter the bloodstream quickly, moderate if they enter at a less rapid rate, and slow when they enter the bloodstream in a relatively slow manner. The glycemic index is derived from comparing all carbs with glucose that has a glycemic index of one hundred.[3] Any carbohydrate with a glycemic index over seventy is considered a high glycemic or "fast" carb, and any below fifty-five are considered slow carbs. Every carb between fifty-five and seventy is considered a moderate carb. So what does this mean for you? It simply means that you should avoid eating fast carbs **exclusively.** Most of the carbs you eat should be of the moderate or slow category in order to keep your insulin response under proper control. Also, when consuming carbs, regardless of their glycemic index, one should always consume an equal caloric amount of protein. I always discuss diet with my patients and it never ceases to amaze me when a patient tells me they are eating in a healthy manner only to find out that they have dry cereal for breakfast, or better yet, a piece of toast and fruit juice. That is the type of misunderstanding that I deal with day in and day out. Those types of meals are essentially all carbs and are simply not healthy.

Patients who eat in that manner have succeeded in doing the one thing they should not do, spiking their insulin and predisposing themselves to a condition known as metabolic syndrome, otherwise known as Syndrome X![4] [5]

Remember, it is high sustained insulin levels that will cause a deterioration of health over time. It doesn't happen overnight; to the contrary, it takes years for insulin dependent diseases to develop and become evident. That is why everyone has heard the story of the person in excellent health that died suddenly of a heart attack. It wasn't sudden; it had been developing for years behind the scenes, same with cancer and stroke. Years of high insulin, because of the intake of fast carbohydrates or a high percentage carb diet, will finally take its toll! Also consider type II diabetes as it can result from the disastrous effect of consuming excessive carbohydrates for many years with the resultant high sustained insulin levels. The American Diabetic Association should be the absolute authority on diet and diabetes, but their recommendation is a diet composed of up to sixty-five percent carbohydrates![6]

Referring back to what I said earlier, low fat or no fat diets **are not healthy**. Consider this: when you reduce the amount of fat in your diet, what are the only two macronutrients that can remain in the food to be consumed? The answer is carbohydrates and proteins. Since carbs are less expensive than proteins as a general rule, most people then choose carbohydrates when they have reduced their fat intake. As a result, a low fat diet becomes a high carbohydrate diet, and that is exactly the type of diet to avoid because of the unwanted high insulin response. The other problem is that many people substitute supposedly bad fats with vegetable oils and margarine (trans-fats).

But insulin is not the only important hormone associated with dietary intake. When one consumes protein, another hormone is secreted called glucagon that helps to control insulin because many of its effects are essentially the opposite of insulin. That is the reason to eat protein with every meal or snack, not to mention the fact that protein is necessary for tissue repair and growth. Protein is composed of amino acids that are the building blocks for muscle and organ tissue. One particular essential amino acid, leucine, has been shown to be a very effective modulator of protein synthesis. Leucine acts as a switch to turn on muscle protein synthesis which in turn requires energy. With a properly balanced diet, stored fat is used for that energy requiring process, ultimately resulting in fat weight loss.[7] If you learn nothing else about diet from this chapter, please remember to always consume protein, including the branched chain amino acid leucine, with carbs and fat at every meal. Unopposed or exclusive carbohydrates are the incorrect way to eat, because they will raise your insulin to higher than needed levels or levels that should never be attained. Doing this infrequently is rarely a problem; however, the danger arises when this habit becomes commonplace and one maintains high insulin levels on a consistent basis. That is one of the suggested contributing factors as to why the otherwise healthy individual dies of cancer or of a previously undiagnosed cardiac event or stroke. For my patients, I recommend reading the books of **Dr. Barry Sears (The Zone series of books)**[8] or the books by **Drs. Mary Dan and Michael Eades starting with Protein Power.**[9] These books provide information that is based upon scientific research instead of unscientific political or business propaganda books written by the "low fat" experts.

What are some examples of foods that are known to be "fast" carbohydrates (carbs) so that you can avoid or reduce them? When patients ask me this question, I always tell them that they don't have to avoid fast carbs, they should simply limit them and always balance them with protein and fat. Some examples of fast carbs are:

- white or whole wheat bread
- taco shells
- pasta
- pastries
- chips
- rice
- rice cakes
- noodles
- dry cereal
- bananas
- fruit juice
- carrots
- potatoes
- corn
- most candy
- cake
- alcoholic beverages
- soft drinks
- low fat ice cream

One ingredient that is often overlooked is high fructose corn syrup. One would think that fructose is good sugar to consume since it is supposedly derived from fruit. Nothing could be further from the truth because fructose should be avoided if possible. For example, sucrose (table sugar) is composed of fifty percent glucose and fifty percent fructose. High fructose corn syrup is fifty-five percent fructose and forty-five percent glucose. The glucose portion of both compounds is not the problem; it is the fructose that is unhealthy because of how it is processed. Even though fructose is not a high glycemic index carbohydrate, it is quite difficult for the liver to metabolize. Because the chemical reaction is so delayed, much of the fructose is converted to fat that is stored in the liver where it is released into the blood stream as triglycerides! That illustrates one of the peculiarities that contradict the erroneous theory that eating fat causes increased fats in the blood. Fructose will result in increased fatty deposits in the belly, thighs, hips, and arms. Unfortunately, high fructose corn syrup is an ingredient in many foods and drinks simply because it is cheap. Sucrose and high fructose corn syrup have contributed to the explosion of obesity in this country. The most prudent course to follow is to become proactive and avoid consuming both. There is absolutely no advantage to consuming fructose; to the contrary, it can definitely result in health issues. Learn to read labels because it is an ingredient in many foods and beverages, including soft drinks. Many weight loss programs have been sabotaged by consuming unsuspected substances such as sucrose or high fructose corn syrup. If you are trying to lose weight or maintain your weight at a certain level, I would also suggest reducing the intake of the previously noted "fast" carb foods or stopping them altogether. Another substance that should be avoided is aspartame, not only because of its toxicity, but because it stimulates the appetite that can result in weight gain.

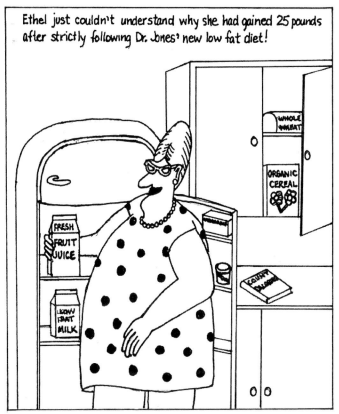

I have many patients who started a dietary program by eliminating all carbohydrates, but I think that is too drastic. Most people who started in that manner will tell you that their energy levels declined severely and that they simply did not feel good for the first three to four days. After that, the body adjusts, but most reach the point of not wanting to continue because it really gets difficult eating just protein and fat without any carbs. If one can tolerate such a diet, it might be a good way to "kick-start" a change in the way they eat, but I would not recommend continuing such a way of eating. Most people who choose that type of diet tend to rebound and gain all weight back, plus more. In many cases, it illustrates the so-called "yo-yo effect" of losing weight and then gaining it back.

If one chooses to begin in that manner, I would suggest adding slow (excluding fructose) or moderate carbs at the end of the first week. Keep in mind that I recommend removing fast carbs from your diet for the first three to four weeks. Once past that point, one may add fast carbs sparingly and just on an intermittent basis and only when counterbalanced by an adequate amount of protein. The reason is the inescapable fact that fast carbs will increase your insulin levels quicker than anything else, and remember that high insulin levels are not in your best interest, health-wise or weight-wise. If one truly wishes to lose fat weight, it is virtually impossible to do so if one continues eating fast carbs as a regular part of one's diet, and believe it or not, adding good fat to a diet helps one lose fat weight.

In the 1990s, another class of carbohydrates was discovered, the eight essential carbohydrates. When I was in medical school, I learned about glycoproteins and their importance in cellular function since they constituted the structure of the cell receptor sites. We knew there were essential amino acids, but at the time, we were not aware that the "glycol" part of the molecule was composed of a certain arrangement of the recently discovered essential carbohydrates. When they are deficient in the diet, then proper receptor site formation is impaired. When the receptor sites are deficient, then the cell reaction mediated by that receptor site doesn't take place. When the body is given an adequate supply of the essential sugars, providing a patient is not protein deficient, the body is able to create the needed receptor sites. The problem that has arisen is the fact that the essential sugars are not plentiful in most diets. With a diet deficient in essential sugars, diseases begin to appear that would not occur otherwise. When receptor sites form without interference, proper health will be maintained as long as other factors are controlled. Even though these are dietary carbohydrates, they are not consumed in sufficient quantity to significantly change the insulin response. The eight essential sugars are: glucose, mannose, fucose, galactose, xylose, N-acetyl galactosamine, N-acetyl glucosamine, and N-acetyl neuraminic acid.

You may also start a change of diet program with a thirty-six hour fast. A fast is exactly what it says, fast! You consume no food and drink, only distilled water. Distilled water is best, but regular filtered tap water is acceptable. Fasting has been looked at as something engaged in by crackpots, but again, the medical profession has probably been wrong. Many books have been written on the subject of fasting. Of course, be sure to consult with a trusted and unbiased physician before considering a fast.

Vegetarians have a more difficult time consuming enough protein simply because most protein is derived from animal sources. Vegans are those people who choose to not consume any protein that is derived from an animal source, so they must get their protein from plant sources such as nuts, beans, soy, or wheat-based products. It can be done, but it is a somewhat more difficult a process. Other vegetarians refrain from eating all meat products except those derived from the water (fish and other types of sea animals).

The majority of people are non-vegetarians who consume all types of protein and have less difficulty finding adequate sources of protein since they also have the choice of beef, pork, chicken, and/or other animal protein. Regardless of the protein source, one needs to consume adequate protein with each meal or snack. As I often tell my patients, if you have a snack without protein, what is left? Of course the answer is either carbohydrates or fats. You already understand what unopposed carbohydrates do to your system, so it is logical to simply not engage in snacking or eating unopposed carbs. Therefore, always eat some type of protein with every snack or meal. The amount of protein one should eat depends upon his or her activity level and whether or not thyroid function is optimal. If you are the type individual who exercises vigorously on a daily basis, then your protein requirement will be much higher than a person who would be considered a "couch potato." For the person who exercises daily and is serious about getting benefit from that exercise, then it is not unrealistic for them to require up to one gram of protein per day for each pound of body weight. However, that requirement is typically too high for people who do not engage in some form of regular exercise. A more exact formula for that requirement of protein can be found in **"The Zone" by Dr. Barry Sears or "Protein Power" by Dr. Eades.** Once you have determined your daily requirement for protein, then you may divide that requirement among your meals and snacks, and remember that every meal or snack should include part of your requirement for protein. After that, the rest is fairly simple as you match the caloric amount of slow or moderate glycemic carbs and fat so that it equals the amount of protein you consume with each meal or snack. Meals should never be spaced more than four to six hours apart with snacks between meals.

I have treated a number of obese individuals during my many years in practice. Of course, each one of them was checked for metabolic issues, particularly hypothyroidism. One thing that I have observed about those patients was that most ate no breakfast! That's a personal observation that I have made, and as you may have guessed by looking at the results, it is a mistake. Avoiding breakfast gets your day off to a bad start provided you're not in the middle of a three day fast as previously mentioned. However, if you have not been eating breakfast, then you need to start, but remember to maintain a balance between the caloric intake of carbs, protein, and fats. In other words, all meals and snacks should be as close to a calorie ratio of 33-33-33% as possible. According to Dr. Barry Sears, one can consume a slightly higher ratio of carbs to protein and still remain in the Zone, but the percentage should never be above a 4:3 ratio of carbs to protein. One can't always be precise, but one should try to maintain that ratio or equal caloric amounts of each. Once you begin to understand caloric balancing, you will be able to adjust your eating habits very easily until it simply becomes a good habit. Keep in mind that calories from protein and carbohydrates are the same, one gram of either a carbohydrate or protein equals four calories. You also must understand that the amount of calories from one gram of fat is more at nine calories per gram. So if you consume one gram of fat, remember that you are ingesting over twice the number of calories compared to the same weight of protein or carbs. Accordingly, that will help you adjust the amount of fat that you will consume to maintain the ratio previously mentioned.

That leads us to the subject of fats. There are a number of books written about the subject of fats. If you read the real science, you will find they are not the villains that many people (doctors) would have you believe. It is very common for patients to tell me that their family doctor or other specialist doctors had told them to avoid eating animal fats or foods containing cholesterol. Simply put, that is mis-information because it is not correct! Unfortunately, many supposedly reliable sources about dietary recommendations are not as reliable as one would believe. A good example is the government sponsored "food pyramid." It was an absolute disaster and was essentially upside down. It has been adjusted recently to reflect some changes, but it is still wrong. I remember when coconut oil and palm oil were used to make popcorn in theaters. Government pressure was brought to bear because those oils were considered dangerous to our health; at least, that was the rationale used. Those very healthy oils were replaced by man-made vegetable oils (including margarine) with resulting molecular structures that had been altered by intense heat and pressure, the so-called trans-fatty acids. Trans-fatty acids are not exactly high on my list of healthy fats and it is ironic that our own government placed pressure on food manufacturers to replace perfectly good health-promoting fats (coconut and palm oil) with fats that are not healthy and possibly more dangerous than we suspect. When things of this nature take place, one should begin looking at the money trail! I was under the impression that our government's main function was to serve and protect us, the citizens! My advice is to avoid trans-fatty acids when possible. How does one do that? **Read labels!** Anything that says "partially hydrogenated" means that it is a trans-fatty acid. Labels can be purposely misleading and rely upon the perception of the customer to sell their unhealthy trans-fatty acid products. Margarine is an example of a trans-fatty acid product that is supposedly healthier than butter, but that is simply untrue. All the beautifully labeled vegetable oils are also trans-fatty acids unless they were **cold-pressed.** Cold-pressed is a term that means that the oil was expressed without the need of heat and high pressure. Virgin olive oil is an example of oil that is made by using the cold press method.

Most have heard that butter and lard are very unhealthy fats, but that is simply not true either. Both can be used without any particular risk because both are saturated. Saturated simply means that the molecule is stable and can't be changed by high heat or pressure. The molecule remains the same as opposed to many other fats that can undergo an unhealthy transformation when exposed to high heat and pressure.

Fish oil is something most people have heard about through commercials or have read about in magazines. Fish oil is composed of omega-3 fatty acids such as DHA (docosahexaenoic acid) and EPA (eicosapentaenoic acid). Both are instrumental in helping form so-called good eiconsanoids and reducing inflammation. Remember that term? They are the short acting very powerful hormone-like substances that have such an impact on your health. Proper intake of omega-3 fatty acids has shown promise in preventing some cancers, probably as a result of modulation of eicosanoids and their associated ability to reduce inflammation. Some eicosanoids are very protective, such as those that promote protection of the stomach lining, while others are not protective and can be detrimental. The balance of eicosanoids is determined strictly by one's diet. Insulin has a damaging effect as it promotes the diversion of the eicosanoid pathway in the wrong direction.

Instead of producing so-called "good" eicosanoids, the body produces eicosanoids like prostaglandins that can result in health issues. There are a number of prostaglandins and within that group are those that can cause joint and muscle pain. In the majority of cases, most people would rather take an anti-inflammatory drug rather than altering their diet. Anti-inflammatory drugs act by reducing the production of eicosanoids, good and bad. Limiting the production of the bad eicosanoids that result in pain is worthwhile, but when the protective hormones (good eicosanoids) are also eliminated, that's when the problems can occur. An example is the person who takes non-steroidal anti-inflammatory drugs (NSAIDs) for joint or muscle pain only to end up with a stomach ulcer with blood loss because the protective mechanism for the stomach lining was also affected. There is much more information about this subject in Dr. Sears' and Dr. Eades books, but suffice it to say that non-steroidal anti-inflammatory drugs should be used sparingly, if at all. Examples of NSAIDs are Motrin®, Naprosyn®, Celebrex®, etc. Aspirin is another anti-inflammatory drug that interferes with the production of eicosanoids. Keep in mind that some eicosanoids can cause problems such thromboxane that promotes platelet adhesion and vasoconstriction. Many doctors recommend taking a daily aspirin in order to reduce the risk of clot formation that could lead to a heart attack. In fact, with the proper alteration of one's diet, the same results could be accomplished as taking an aspirin a day. However, our medical culture is based upon taking a pill and treating symptoms instead of preventing the symptoms.

Water is very important in the overall equation for optimum health. The human body is composed primarily of water, and in order to maintain a proper balance, sufficient quantities of water should be consumed daily. Most authentic experts agree that eight ounces of water eight times per day is the minimum amount necessary to prevent dehydration and provide sufficient volume for many body functions and chemical reactions necessary for optimum health. The portable water industry has taken advantage of this need and a multi-billion dollar plus industry was created by selling us water in plastic bottles. Some of the water sold is simply filtered and not pure spring water as the label may imply. My greatest concern about bottled water is the *plastic bottles* that contain the water. Plastics are not meant to be consumed; to the contrary, plastics are very unhealthy and should not be consumed. In order to make plastics more soft and pliable, compounds known as phthalates are used. More and more information is being made available about the toxicity of phthalates, but we continue drinking water from plastic bottles containing those toxic chemicals. Heating those bottles causes the release of more phthalates. Unfortunately, phthalates are used in many things including hair sprays, some cosmetics, toys, colognes, and wood finishers. That "new car" smell is the pungent odor of phthalates that is even more evident when the outside temperature is high. As the temperature goes down, the phthalates condense and form an oily film on the inside of windshields. So why the concern? We know that higher doses are associated with cancer and adult infertility, but it is the low dose toxicity that has caused concern. We now have evidence that low dose phthalates can cause serious problems with the developing male fetus, as well as early sexual maturation of pre-pubescent females.[10] Perhaps it would be more advisable to simply filter water at home and work and drink the water from a glass container. That would not eliminate phthalates, but it would be a start.

Notes

[1] Keys A., "Seven Countries: A multivariate analysis of death and coronary heart disease." Harvard University Press, 1980; Cambridge MA.

[2] Shaw I., *The Oxford History of Ancient Egypt*, Oxford University Press, 2000.

[3] Jenkins D.J. et al, "Glycemic index of foods, a physiologic basis for carbohydrate exchange." *American Journal of Clinical Nutrition*, 1981; 34:362-366.

[4] Sears B., *Enter The Zone*, 1995; "The Zone and Your Heart." 13:146.

[5] Reaven G.M. et al, "Abnormalities of carbohydrate metabolism my play a role in the etiology and clinical course of hypertension." *Trends in Pharmacolical Science*. 1998; 9:78-79.

[6] Katsilambros, M. et al, "Critical Review of the international guidelines:what is agreed upon-what is not?" Nestle Nutr Workshop Ser Clin Perform Program, 2006; 11:207-218.

[7] Layman, D.K, "The role of leucine in weight loss diets and glucose homeostasis." *Journal of Nutrition*, 2003;133:261S-267S.

[8] Sears, Barry et al, *Enter The Zone*. New York: Harper Collins, 1995. Print. *The Anti-Aging Zone*. New York: Harper Collins, 1999. Print. *A Week In The Zone*. New York: Harper Collins. 2000. Print.

[9] Eades, M.R. & M.D. *Protein Power*. New York: Bantam Books. 1996. Print.

[10] Tilson H.A., "EHP Papers of the Year, 2008." Environ. Health Perspect., June 2008; 116(6):A234.

7

MICRONUTRIENTS AND MORE

Many volumes of work have been written and published about vitamins and minerals (micronutrients). Since this chapter is not intended to answer every question about these ubiquitous substances, additional information is readily available in libraries. Medical training for doctors provides only basic information about the subject. Everything learned after that point results from independent investigation. Accordingly, it is logical to assume that many doctors know very little about the subject of micronutrients. One needs to understand that a proper diet supplies some of our requirement for micronutrients, but supplementation is indicated when that requirement is not met. When supplementing, it is important to understand that a vitamin or mineral supplement is no better than its ability to be absorbed. A number of highly visible and well known supplement brands have poor qualities of absorption. It should be noted that there are two diametrically opposed viewpoints on the subject of micronutrients. At one end of the spectrum is the group that makes the claim that no supplementation is necessary because the diet supplies us with the micronutrients necessary for good health. An example of this faulty argument is the essential element iodine that was discussed in the chapter on hypothyroidism. If we were to believe the group (endocrinologists) that recommends restricting our intake of iodine to 0.2 mg per day, the result would be a population deficient in iodine. Unfortunately, that seems to have already taken place as the extremists on that end of the spectrum hold positions of power and influence that, in turn, have shaped the opinions of the populace in regard to iodine. At the other end of the spectrum is the group that recommends mega-dosing most micronutrients. Where does the truth lie? As with most things, the truth lies somewhere in the middle because critical thinking is absent in both groups. When science becomes politicized, opinions should always be suspect.

There are micronutrients that are supplied by the diet, but there are also those that must be supplemented. Vitamin C is an example of a water soluble vitamin that must be supplied as the human body can't manufacture it. The B-complex vitamins are also water soluble. Any excess water soluble vitamin is typically eliminated by the kidneys and is not stored for extended periods. However, there are side effects of consuming excessive amounts. In the case of fat soluble vitamins such as A, D, E, and K, consuming excessive amounts will result in the storage of those particular vitamins in fatty tissue and the liver. An excess level of any vitamin is referred to as hypervitaminosis. The condition occurs primarily with the fat soluble vitamins for the reasons noted. How dangerous is hypervitaminosis and in which age group does it typically occur? The symptoms are varied and depend on the vitamin ingested. It is extremely rare for anyone to die as the result of hypervitaminosis and about eighty percent of all cases occur in children under the age of six.[1] When hypervitaminosis occurs, it is always labeled with the vitamin involved. As an example, hypervitaminosis C is the name given to excessive levels of vitamin C. The condition can result in diarrhea, but every individual's tolerance level is different. When the intake of vitamin C is stopped or reduced, the symptoms resolve quickly.

Vitamin C

It is known that the requirement for vitamin C is increased in certain disease states; therefore, one can titrate (gradually increase) the dose of vitamin C upward until symptoms of diarrhea begin (titrating to bowel tolerance).[2] Vitamin C is very important in the healing process and I typically recommend 2,000-3,000 milligrams per day for patients undergoing prolotherapy, for patients who have sustained injuries, or those who are attempting to recuperate from an illness. Vitamin C is of utmost importance in the formation of collagen that is a component in every support structure in the body such as tendons, ligaments, muscle tissue, vessels, joint capsules, internal organs, and skin. Accordingly, a deficiency of vitamin C can result in scurvy, because of the disruption of collagen formation, with its attendant easy bruising of the skin, anemia, weakness, fatigue, low blood pressure, chest pain, and joint pain.

Vitamin B

The B vitamins are designated by a number after the "B." Accordingly, there are eight "B" vitamins beginning with thiamine or B1. The other seven B vitamins are B2 (riboflavin), B3 (niacin), B5 (pantothenic acid), B6 (pyridoxine), B7 (biotin), B9 (folic acid), and B12 (cobalamins). There are obvious "gaps" within the numbering system for the B vitamins. That occurred because of past identification errors wherein various non-vitamin substances had been initially identified as a "B" vitamin. For example, adenine was considered a B vitamin for a period of time and was given the label vitamin B4. However, that label was removed when it was discovered that adenine was not truly a vitamin, but an integral molecule involved in the formation of DNA. Similar identification problems occurred with a number of other molecules that were labeled as B vitamins initially, up to and including vitamin B22. "B" vitamins promote a number of functions in the human body including the maintenance of an optimal metabolic rate. That is achieved primarily with vitamin B12 because it is involved in the conversion of T4 to T3. The B vitamins help maintain healthy skin and muscle tone. They also promote proper immune function, cell division, and proper functioning of the nervous system. Those are some of the general functions that are assisted by the B complex vitamins.

More specifically, a lack of any of the B complex vitamins can result in specific conditions. With severe chronic deficiencies of B1 and B3, the end result can be death. A condition known as beriberi results from a lack of B1. The symptoms of beriberi are related to the destabilization of the nervous system and may include emotional disturbances, weakness and pain in the limbs, weak heart beat, and swelling of the hands and feet. Vitamin B2 deficiency is characterized by sensitivity to sunlight, cracking of the lips, sore throat, inflammation of the tongue, and dermatitis. The condition resulting from a deficiency of B3 is called pellegra and the symptoms are confusion, dermatitis, aggression, weakness, and diarrhea. B5 deficiency can result in acne and paresthesias (tingling, numbness) in the hands and feet. A lack of vitamin B6 can cause high blood pressure, dermatitis, depression, swelling, anemia, and an elevation of homocysteine. Some believe that elevated homocysteine levels are a risk factor for heart disease, but that hypothesis is still being studied. B7 deficiency rarely causes any problems in adults, but can affect infants by retarding growth and the maturation of the nervous system. Vitamin B9 (folic acid) deficiency can cause macrocytic anemia and high levels of the amino acid homocysteine. A deficiency of B9 also increases the risk of birth defects, so it is recommended that all pregnant women take folic acid in appropriate doses. Vitamin B12 deficiency can result in macrocytic anemia, fatigue, peripheral neuropathies, memory loss, and difficulty concentrating. Vegetarians should take a B12 supplement since there is little to no B12 in vegetables. Like vitamin C, the B vitamins are water soluble and any excess is typically excreted through the kidneys. Toxicity can occur if one consumes excessive quantities of water soluble vitamins, but it is rare since they are typically not stored. While toxicity is uncommon, excessive doses of B3 can result in nausea, vomiting, and flushing of the skin. Excessive B6 can result in painful peripheral neuropathies (painful extremities with associated tingling/numbness). B9 is not toxic, but it can result in masking the symptoms of B12 deficiency. A well absorbed B complex vitamin complex, in tablet or capsule form, typically provides enough of each of the B vitamins for a healthy adult.

Vitamin A

Vitamin A is a fat soluble vitamin best known for its role in assisting with vision, particularly low light and color vision. One often associates vitamin A with carrots because carrots have the highest vitamin A concentration of any vegetable or fruit. However, the highest concentration is found in the liver of beef, chicken, pork, fish, turkey, and cod liver oil. Vitamin A also functions in assisting gene transcription (activation). It also is involved in the immune and the hemopoietic (blood) systems as it plays a role in the differentiation of blood cells starting with stem cells found in the bone marrow. Vitamin A is also a known antioxidant and it helps in bone maturation, epithelial cell development, and the healing response.

As with any vitamin, either a deficiency or excess can result in problems. Vitamin A deficiency is estimated to affect approximately one third of children worldwide under the age of five.[3] Out of the children affected annually by vitamin A deficiency, it has been further estimated to claim 670,000 lives.[4] Another estimated 250,000 to 500,000 children in the same group go blind each year because of deficiency of vitamin A.[5] Vitamin A deficiency happens in two ways. The first is due to the lack of ingested vitamin A due to starvation or inadequate supply of foods containing the vitamin. A deficiency can also result from the inability to absorb fats, and since vitamin A is fat soluble, the process becomes impaired. It is also known that reduced absorption of vitamin A is related to alcoholism and cigarette smoking. Regardless of the mechanism of how vitamin A deficiency occurs, the most usual early sign of deficiency is night blindness or the inability to see when less light is available. It is an insidious process as one's inability to see at night progresses to gradually requiring more and more light to see. If not detected and left untreated, the condition can progressively worsen with severe dryness of the eyes that can cause damage to the cornea with end stage blindness. As noted previously, vitamin A is also necessary for proper immune function, and a deficiency can result in impairment after which the host becomes susceptible to a myriad of infections.

It is much more difficult for the body to eliminate fat soluble vitamins as compared to the water soluble vitamins. As a result of staying in the system for longer periods of time, the fat soluble vitamins, including vitamin A, are more prone to cause toxicity if excessive amounts are ingested. Toxicity from vitamin A is characterized by nausea, vomiting, blurred vision, anorexia, irritability, hair loss, muscle pain and weakness, mental confusion, drowsiness, insomnia, fatigue, and weight loss. There have been reports of excess vitamin A causing osteoporosis, but the studies include other variables that may have been more responsible.[6] I typically recommend for adults to take no more than 3,000 micrograms of Vitamin A per day.

Vitamin E

Vitamin E is another fat soluble vitamin and one that I advise patients to take for its antioxidant capabilities. Vitamin E is the common name given to a group of eight compounds known as tocopherols and tocotrienols. There are four each of each group that are designated by "alpha, beta, gamma, and delta." The "alpha" form of the tocopherol is the most studied and well known of the vitamin E group, and is the only one of the eight known to be required by the human body. However, that assumption may be based upon the fact that the other seven known E vitamins have not been studied to any great extent. Alpha tocopherol is known to have antioxidant capabilities by acting as a "scavenger" of free radicals that cause cell damage and may contribute to the development of cardiovascular disease and cancer.[7] Free radicals can result from exposure to ultraviolet radiation from the sun, smoking, and air pollution. When free radicals react with oxygen, the result is the formation of reactive oxygen species (ROS). Vitamin E interferes with the formation of

ROS when fat undergoes oxidation. Vitamin E also plays a role in the immune function, cell signaling, and the regulation of gene expression. Vitamin E helps the interior of blood vessels to remain more resistant to the adhesion of blood cell components and reduces platelet adhesion, resulting in a lesser tendency to clot prematurely or needlessly. Accordingly, there is evidence that vitamin E is important in reducing the incidence of heart attacks,[8] although additional studies about this subject are needed. Unfortunately, evidence is inconsistent and limited about whether or not vitamin E is helpful in preventing cancer. The same holds true for vitamin E preventing age-related macular degeneration and cataracts. The evidence is not convincing, but the use of vitamin E is probably just one part of the puzzle. It has also been suggested that vitamin E is helpful in reducing the incidence of mental decline seen with aging. More research about the role of vitamin E for cognitive disorders is needed.

Deficiency of vitamin E is rare, but when it occurs, symptoms may include peripheral neuropathies, impaired immune function, retinopathy, muscle weakness, and ataxia (impaired muscle control). Since vitamin E is a fat soluble vitamin, it requires the presence of fat for absorption. In conditions that interfere with absorption, such as Crohn's disease, liver disease, and cystic fibrosis, a water soluble form of vitamin E may have to be substituted. As with any fat soluble vitamin, toxicity can develop when excess vitamin E is consumed on a chronic basis. It has been suggested that excessive vitamin E results the interruption of normal blood coagulation by interfering with platelet aggregation. Platelets are an integral and necessary component of clotting and when that is impaired, abnormal and extended bleeding can occur.

Information regarding safe doses of vitamin E is limited due to the fact that vitamin E has been studied less than most other vitamins. It has been suggested that the top safe level for vitamin E is 1,500 IUs in adults. One must exercise caution with taking vitamin E if they are taking an antiplatelet or anticoagulant such as Coumadin because it can potentiate the risk of bleeding.

Vitamin D

Vitamin D is the general term for another group of fat soluble vitamins. When discussing vitamin D, I will be referring to the two important forms, D2 and D3. Ultraviolet B light from the sun results in the production of vitamin D in the skin. Food sources rich in vitamin D are fatty fish, meats, and eggs. Vitamin D can also be consumed as a capsule or tablet. Vitamin D is transported through the blood stream to the liver where it is converted to the metabolite calcidiol (D2) that is then converted into the physiologically active vitamin D metabolite, calcitriol (D3). In the active state, vitamin D is involved in the regulation of a number of body functions including the maintenance of proper bone mineralization by stabilizing proper levels of phosphate and calcium in the blood. It also plays a significant role in maximizing many components of the immune system with its obvious role of keeping the body free of infection. Vitamin D also influences genes responsible for cellular proliferation, differentiation, and apoptosis (death).[9]

Deficiency of vitamin D is best known for causing rickets. Rickets is a childhood disease characterized by impaired growth and deformity of the long bones of the upper and lower extremities.[10] Vitamin D deficiency is not the only cause of rickets, but it is the most widely known. Osteomalacia or bone thinning is another condition caused by vitamin D deficiency. It is typically associated with proximal muscle weakness and bone fragility. It has been reported that vitamin D deficiency is also associated with peripheral vascular disease (hardening of the arteries), multiple sclerosis, rheumatoid arthritis, type I diabetes, Parkinson's disease, Alzheimer's disease, and some forms of cancer.[11] [12] In view of the role of vitamin D in the maintenance of healthy hair follicles, a deficiency could result in hair loss.

As with many subjects in nutrition, there is controversy regarding whether or not most people need to supplement with oral forms of vitamin D. For normal fair-skinned individuals, exposure to the sun or ultraviolet light for about twenty minutes a day allows enough vitamin D production to reach equilibrium and any further production is degraded and excreted. Individuals with a higher degree of pigmentation in the skin (darker-skinned) require three to six times longer exposure to reach the same equilibrium. If an individual remains exposed to ultraviolet B rays long enough, sunburn will begin to occur. That is referred to as an "erythemal dose" and exposure of that type will result in the production of between 10,000 to 25,000 IUs of vitamin D depending upon the individual.[13] Regardless of how much an individual is exposed to UV light or the sun, there is no known toxicity from vitamin D formed in the skin.[14] With the discovery of how much vitamin D the skin can produce, some have recommended that the upper tolerable daily intake of vitamin D be raised to 10,000 IUs.[15] However, there is a difference in the manner in which sunlight derived (endogenous) vitamin D is used by the body as compared to that which is supplemented (exogenous).[16] Therein lies the basis for the controversy concerning how much vitamin D that individuals can safely take. Everyone is different because of genetics, environmental factors, and dietary regimen. For example, if a fair-skinned individual is exposed to sunlight on a regular basis, the need for vitamin D supplementation is typically not an issue. Darker skinned individuals tend to not form as much vitamin D in the skin and that factor would have to be considered if the question was raised about supplementing with vitamin D. The same would hold true for individuals whose life style kept them out of the sun. For those over the age of nine that require vitamin D supplementation, I recommend taking no more than 5,000 IUs per day. That amount is twenty-five percent higher than the recommended upper tolerable limit suggested by the Institute of Medicine.

For patients under the age of nine, I concur with the recommendations set by the Institute of Medicine, wherein the recommendation is no more than 1,000 IUs for infants up to one year of age, 2,500 IUs for children ages one through three, and 3,000 IUs for ages four through eight.[17] The research is ongoing in this interesting area and that may result in changes for the suggested upper tolerable limits. Toxicity can occur when vitamin D is consumed in larger doses, but that dose is significantly higher than what I recommend and what is recommended by the Institute of Medicine. Studies have shown that healthy adults taking 50,000 IUs for several months can develop toxicity.[18] The underlying cause of toxicity to vitamin D is hypercalcemia (excessive calcium in the blood). The initial symptoms are nausea, vomiting, and anorexia (loss of appetite). If left undiagnosed, those symptoms can be followed by polydipsia (excessive thirst), polyuria (excessive urination), prutitis (itching), anxiety, and weakness. Untreated hypercalcemia can lead to renal failure that is often irreversible. Pregnant women should consult with their doctor before taking higher doses of vitamin D, as toxicity can result in mental retardation and facial deformities in the unborn fetus. Accordingly, it is advisable to exercise caution and avoid taking high levels of vitamin D for extended periods. It is rare that toxicity develops, but if it should, the treatment is to stop all vitamin D supplementation and restrict calcium intake. Generally speaking, either a deficiency or an excess of vitamin D can result in abnormal function and premature aging.[19] Based upon the available data, it is probable that there is a narrow range in which vitamin D promotes optimal metabolic function.

Vitamin K

Vitamin K is the general term for another group of fat soluble vitamins, but the current thinking is that only vitamin K1 (phylloquinone) and vitamin K2 (menaquinone) are important in humans. As with the other vitamins, the vitamins K are still being studied and some functions remain unknown.

However, we do know that vitamins K are important for proper clotting of the blood and bone metabolism. Those taking Coumadin must realize that taking vitamin K1 or K2 supplements may interfere with that medication.[20] Vitamin K2 is not affected by aspirin, in contrast to vitamin K1. As with discussion of most vitamins, there is controversy concerning whether or not humans should supplement with vitamins K. In the past, the concept was that everyone absorbed sufficient amounts unless the intestines were damaged and unable to absorb vitamins K. We now believe that they are not that well absorbed from the intestines even when functioning normally.[21] In order to ensure proper levels of vitamins K, it has been suggested that supplementation may be indicated. The recommended dose of vitamins K is 120 micrograms for adult males and ninety micrograms for adult females. Up to 1,000 micrograms per day may be needed for optimal bone metabolism.[22] While deficiency can occur, it is very rare in healthy adults. Deficiencies are more commonly seen in infants, particularly those born prematurely, and individuals with liver damage or disease, cystic fibrosis, inflammatory bowel disease, Crohn's disease, ulcerative colitis, and those who have undergone recent abdominal surgery. Secondary deficiencies can result from those on stringent diets, on anticoagulants, or those with eating disorders such as anorexia and bulimia. Symptoms of deficiency include easy bruising, anemia, bleeding of the gums or nose, and heavy menstrual periods in women. Osteoporosis and coronary artery disease are also strongly associated with lower levels of vitamin K2. In contrast to other fat soluble vitamins, there seems to be no toxicity to high doses of either vitamin K1 or K2. However, a synthetic form of vitamin K, menadione (K3), is very toxic when taken in large doses.

A number of other "micronutrients" are necessary for continuing optimum health and function. They are referred to as minerals, when in fact that label is somewhat misleading. A more appropriate term is **chemical elements**, but the term "mineral" has been so widely used that it simply becomes an exercise in semantics. There are four basic elements inherent in all living organisms, oxygen, nitrogen, carbon and hydrogen, but those will not be part of the discussion even though they are definitely essential for life. There are sixteen additional minerals that are derived from a proper diet, but each can be supplemented in case of deficiencies. Seven of the sixteen are considered "quantity" chemical elements simply because a greater amount of each is necessary in order to assure proper functioning of the body processes. The remaining nine are considered "trace" elements because the amount required of each is much less than the quantity elements.

The quantity elements are sodium, potassium, chlorine, magnesium, calcium, phosphorus, and sulfur. Their necessity is the result of each being involved in chemical processes or by becoming an integral part of the formation of body structures. **Sodium** is an electrolyte that plays a pivotal role in cellular function by co-regulating cellular metabolism with potassium for the creation of energy. Dietary sources of sodium are table salt, sea vegetables, spinach, and dairy products. **Potassium** is also an electrolyte that, as indicated, works in conjunction with sodium to co-regulate cellular metabolism. Examples of dietary sources for potassium include bananas, tomatoes, potato skins, and legumes. **Chlorine** is another electrolyte derived primarily from table salt, but is also found in a number of fruits and vegetables and is used in the production of stomach acid (hydrochloric acid) for digestion. It also plays a role in the maintenance of a proper body pH and assists with cellular metabolism along with sodium and potassium. **Magnesium** is essential for forming healthy bones and is also involved in the process of creating cellular energy. Dietary sources of magnesium are nuts, soy beans, and cocoa. **Calcium** is important for proper health of muscles, the heart, and the digestive system. It is also involved in the synthesis and function of blood cells and the formation and maintenance of bone. Typical dietary sources are dairy products, nuts, seeds, green leafy vegetables, salmon, and sardines. **Phosphorus** is also an important component of energy production and is an integral part of the structure of bone and teeth in conjunction with calcium. It assists with proper function of the muscles and heart and optimizes nerve conduction and kidney function. In order to ensure proper bone mineralization, it is important to take both calcium and phosphorus. Phosphorus is present in many foods and a deficiency is quite rare. **Sulfur** is used primarily in the formation of some amino acids that subsequently combine to form proteins. It is a necessary component in the structure of cells. A deficiency of sulfur is very rare, particularly if one eats a balanced diet and has no problems with absorption.

The trace chemical elements are iodine, zinc, iron, manganese, copper, selenium, molybdenum, cobalt, and nickel. I have seen fluoride described as a trace chemical element, but that is another example of pseudoscience backed by a marketing campaign. *There is absolutely no requirement for fluoride in the proper function and health of the human body.* The only supposed purpose of fluoride is to prevent tooth decay. Fluoride in water does **nothing** to prevent tooth decay; to the contrary, it is only fluoride that is applied topically that shows any reduction in tooth decay. So why is fluoride in our water supply? The decision to place fluoride in the public water supply was made by government bureaucrats who used extremely poor science to justify their stance. Unfortunately, government authorities don't have to answer to the public they are supposed to protect, and removing it from the water supply will be met with bureaucratic red tape. The biggest concern about fluoride is that it resides in the very same category (halides) of the periodic table (grouping of atoms) with an authentic and truly essential chemical element, **iodine.** Because of the similar characteristics, it has been proposed that it competes with iodine for iodine receptor sites and can result in a number of very serious problems if it substitutes for iodine. It's an area of controversy and a number of questions about its use have yet to be answered scientifically. Suffice it to say that the recommended daily allowance is far too low because the estimate was based upon faulty studies and reasoning.

The trace element, **zinc,** is a required factor for many enzymes. It is important for immune function and there is conflicting data that zinc may help reduce symptoms of the common cold. It also assists with proper nerve transmission, protects cell membranes against oxidation, helps to ensure proper gestation, and determines the length of cell life. Zinc is an important component of the healing response as well. The most well known requirement for **iron** is for the production of hemoglobin that allows red blood cells to transport oxygen from the lungs to peripheral tissues. Without iron, a person will develop iron deficient anemia and the supply of oxygen to tissues becomes impaired. Iron is important in the formation of myoglobin that transports oxygen from hemoglobin to muscle cells. It is important in the formation of cytochromes that play a vital role in energy production and also assists in the proper function of the immune system.

Manganese is a cofactor in many enzymatic reactions. It has been postulated that manganese deficiency can lead to osteoporosis. An excess may result in trembling, calf muscle spasm, and impotence. A very serious disorder, similar to Parkinson's with psychiatric and motor disturbances (manganism), can develop from long term exposure to manganese. **Copper** is involved in the formation of cytochrome oxidase protein complex found in mitochondria (energy manufacturing organelles) within cells. Copper also assists in the healing process by helping form cross links within collagen. It has been suggested that copper deficiency is one of the factors leading to the development of coronary artery disease. Toxicity from copper is rare, but is manifested by nausea, vomiting, and muscle pain, and can be relieved by stopping the intake of copper or by increasing the intake of zinc. **Selenium** is best known as an essential cofactor in antioxidant enzymes such as glutathione peroxidase. It is also an important cofactor in the conversion of T4 to T3 (thyroid).

Claims have also been made about the cancer preventing properties of selenium, but the evidence is mixed to support the hypothesis.[23] The recommended daily intake of selenium is about 400 micrograms per day. **Molybdenum** is a component of many enzymes affecting protein synthesis, metabolism and growth. Toxicity is extremely rare in humans. The average daily intake is between 0.12 and 0.24mg per day and toxicity can develop when more than 10mg is consumed per day. The chief cause of deficiency is due to low soil concentration of this trace element. Deficiency of molybdenum is associated with a significantly increased risk of esophageal cancer.[24] **Cobalt** is necessary for the formation of vitamin B12. Although quite rare, a deficiency of cobalt could lead to macrocytic anemia due to impaired synthesis of vitamin B12. **Nickel** is an element present in some enzymes. It is also present in one of the families of superoxide dismutases, but not known to be present in humans.

There are some other substances that deserve mentioning simply because of reports about their use. For sake of brevity, I will mention a few of the more popular names with which the reader may be familiar. **Resveratrol** is a term that most readers are familiar with, but know little about. Resveratrol was actually first written about in 1939, so it is obviously not a recent discovery.[25] A number of controversial claims have been made about resveratrol because the evidence for those claims is conflicting in many cases. For example, a claim has been made that resveratrol improves longevity. The studies about resveratrol and longevity were published in 2003 and concluded that it was indeed effective in extending the lifespan. However, the subjects of the study were not humans, they were *worms and fruit flies*.[26] Proponents of anti-aging took that fact out of context and concluded that it was likewise effective in humans. While there is a possibility, jumping to that conclusion is simply junk science. The only true method of making that determination is to engage in a properly designed study in humans. Until that is accomplished, resveratrol's ability to lengthen the lifespan of humans is merely conjecture and wishful thinking. It has also been touted as an anti-cancer agent; however, similar to the subject of increasing longevity, no studies have been performed in humans. As a result, no conclusions can be legitimately reached about anti-cancer effects in humans. There have also been a number of other noted effects of resveratrol including anti inflammation, anti-diabetes, antivirus, cardioprotection, and neuroprotection. Those results were seen in animal studies and conclusions about its effect in humans can only be speculated. Generally speaking, the positive benefits of resveratrol seem promising, but the mechanism of action in humans has yet to be determined, and the facts about long term usage in humans is unknown. As with any dietary supplement, it is certainly not a panacea for all ills, regardless of the many claims made by promoters.

Another nutritional substance recently in the news has been the **açai** (pronounced ah-sigh-ee) berry. The small, dark purple berry comes from the açai palm tree. A number of claims for the use in humans have been made, but as with resveratrol, the scientific evidence to support those claims has been very limited. It has been touted as a weight loss supplement, but support for that claim has been anecdotal without any explanation concerning the mechanism of action. That does not mean that açai does not assist in weight loss, it simply has not been shown how or why it works scientifically. It may eventually be scientifically determined that açai does indeed work for stimulating weight loss, but that proof is yet to come. One of the reasons why açai became popular was because of promotion through multi-level marketing. Minimal scientific evidence is available to support their claims. There is no evidence that it reverses diabetes or any other chronic medical condition. Claims have also been made that açai promotes restful sleep, improves sexual function, increases energy, and detoxifies the body. To date, none of those claims have been scientifically proven. The açai berry supposedly has the highest antioxidant benefit compared to other foods, but scientific testing actually found that not to be the case.[27] [28]

Coenzyme Q10 (CoQ10) is one of many cofactors necessary for chemical reactions to take place within cells. There are literally hundreds of cofactors that bind with enzymes to increase the rate of a specific chemical reaction. Coenzyme Q10 is being mentioned simply because it has been marketed successfully and is better known than many others. It is also known as ubiquinone, or the more reduced and bio-available form, ubiquinol. It is a fat soluble vitamin-like substance (cofactor) that is present in the mitochondria of all cells with a nucleus (eukaryotic). It functions as a coenzyme for producing energy in the form of ATP. Ninety-five percent of the body's energy is produced in this manner and that fact alone emphasizes the importance of this coenzyme. Organs such as the heart, brain, and kidneys have a very high energy requirement and coenzyme Q10 is found in greater concentration in these organs. It can also function as an important antioxidant, particularly in its reduced form, ubiquinol. CoQ10 can be taken as a supplement, but it is also present in its highest concentrations in organ meats, soy beans, grape seeds, peanuts, sesame seeds, pistachio nuts, avodados, parsley, and spinach. As a supplement, the upper observed safe level (OSL) is 1,200mg per day. There does not seem to be toxicity associated with much higher doses, but some people have reported gastrointestinal problems. The need for CoQ10 is increased in disease states. It has noted to be useful with such conditions as cancer, congestive heart failure, hypertension, migraine headaches, Parkinson's, and cardiac arrest. A study with rats showed an increased lifespan of rats given CoQ10 in comparison with controls receiving no CoQ10. No human studies have been undertaken in that regard.

Another area of interest has been the role played by the **omega-3 fatty acids** (fish oil). Overall, they are part of a class of nutrients known as essential fatty acids that are necessary for life itself. A number of omega-3 fatty acids exist in nature, but three are thought to be the most important. The three are alphalinolenic acid (ALA), eicosapentanoic acid (EPA), and docosapentanoic acid (DHA). Many take fish oil in order to ingest their daily recommendation of omega-3s, but don't understand the exact mechanism as to how they work. The mechanism of action is somewhat complicated. However, I will attempt to simplify the process so the next time one ingests omega-3s, they will understand why. In order to begin the process of understanding omega-3s, one needs to understand the term, eicosanoid. Very simply, an eicosanoid is a short acting hormone made by body cells from omega-6 and omega-3 acids. While omega-3 fatty acids are the basis of some eicosanoids, they are also important for supporting production of so-called "good" eicosanoids and preventing production of "bad" eicosanoids from omega-6 fatty acids. Confused yet? The type of eicosanoid produced is determined by the type diet one eats. There are over a hundred eicosanoids that modulate many body functions such as clotting, healing, inflammation/immune function, maintenance of artery walls, and protection of the stomach lining. Aspirin and the non-steroidal anti-inflammatory drugs (NSAIDs) all work by changing the levels of eicosanoids. The oldest NSAIDs were generalized in their effects and interfered with the synthesis of most eicosanoids. There are eicosanoids that cause pain and inflammation that are classified as protaglandins. When an NSAID is taken, it blocks the synthesis of the pain producing prostaglandin, but unfortunately, it can also block so called "good" eicosanoids such as those that protect the lining of the stomach and intestines. Eicosanoids are actually neither bad nor good, but some are much more beneficial than others and it is wise to maintain a balance of eicosanoids by consuming the proper type of diet. A proper diet is a balanced diet. The diet recommended by the American Diabetic Association is too high in carbohydrates and stimulates elevated insulin levels. In turn, insulin has an impact on the type eicosanoids produced and the results are not favorable. A more appropriate and healthy diet is one that has essentially equal caloric levels of protein, carbohydrates, and fats. When adequate protein is consumed with an equal amount of carbohydrates, the insulin response is more controlled, thereby maintaining a more healthy balance of eicosanoids. I believe that life changing discoveries are yet to made about eicosanoids and how to achieve proper balance throughout life. As a result, I believe that they represent one of the important pieces of the puzzle to promote optimum health and longevity.

Speaking of longevity, a very promising and exciting area of biotechnology exists and has been evolving for about ten years. This new area of cellular biology seems more akin to science fiction than real science. Scientists have known that cells have life spans that are predetermined. Determining why cells live a certain length of time before dying (apoptosis) has been an unanswered question until recently. Cells continue to duplicate themselves by cell division (mitosis) until they reach the point at which the process stops. The question about why the duplication process stops is the key. A component of the cellular duplication process is known as the telomere which is a part of the cellular DNA. It was discovered that the telomere only had a certain length and when the extent of that length was reached, the cell stopped duplicating and died. An enzyme, telomerase, was discovered as the substance that determined telomere length, and ultimately its lifespan.[29] The exciting part of this story is the discovery of the process that lengthens the telomere and extends the life of the cell itself. Theoretically, if the telomere possessed an innate ability to lengthen itself, the cell would become immortal. It holds great promise in extending life, and anti-aging proponents are claiming that this is the next step in understanding why we age. Shortened telomere life is associated with a number of premature aging conditions.[30] While controlling the telomere lifespan holds definite promise in extending healthy life, it is also known to extend the life of unwanted cells. It is exactly the type of process that occurs with cancer cells and one of the reasons why cancer is so difficult to eradicate.[31] The obvious problem associated with the extension of telomere life is, how do we effectively enhance the duplication and longevity of normal cells while protecting against cancer cells? While telomere science is exciting and promising, it is a double-edged sword. Studies are ongoing in this field and many discoveries are yet to come. Could this be the key to extending life and treating many diseases including cancer? Time will tell and volumes will be written about this subject.

Notes

[1] 2004 Annual Report of the American Association of Poison Control Centers Toxic Exposure Surveillance System.

[2] Cathcart, R., "Vitamin C, Titrating to Bowel Tolerance, Anascorbemia and Acute Induced Scurvy," 1994.

[3] World Health Organization, Global prevalence of vitamin A deficiency in populations at risk 1995-2005, WHO global database on vitamin A deficiency.

[4] Black, R.E.; Allen, LH et al; "Maternal and child undernutrition: global and regional exposures and health consequences." Lancet 371 (9608):243-260.

[5] Office of dietary supplements, Vitamin A. National Institute of Health; April 8 2008.

[6] Forsmo, Siri et al; "Childhood Cod Liver Oil Consumption and Bone Mineral Density in a Population-based Cohort of Peri and Postmenopausal Women:The Nord-Trondelag Health Study." Am. J. Epidemiol. 167 (4): 406-411.

[7] Verhagen, H et al The state of antioxidant affairs. Nutrition Today 2006; 41:244-250.

[8] Glynn, RJ et al Effects of random allocation to vitamin E supplementation on the occurrence of venous thromboemobilism: report from the Womens' Health Study. Circulation 2007; 116:1497-1503.

[9] "Dietary Supplement Fact Sheet: Vitamin D." Office of Dietary Supplements. National Institutes of Health.

[10] Lerch, C. et al "Interventions for the prevention of nutritional rickets in term born children." Cochrane database for systematic reviews (Online) (4): CD006164.

[11] Holick, M.F., "Sunlight and vitamin D for bone health and prevention of autoimmune diseases, cancers and cardiovascular disease." The American Journal of Clinical Nutrition; 2004:80(6 Suppl.) 1678-1688.

[12] Evatt, ML et al, "Prevalence of vitamin D insufficiency in patients with Parkinson disease and Alzheimer disease." Archives of Neurology; 65(10) 1348-1352.

[13] Holick, M.F., "Environmental factors that influence the cutaneous production of vitamin D." The American Journal of Clinical Nutrition; March 1995:61 (3 suppl.) 638-645.

[14] Vieth, R. "Vitamin D supplementation, 25-hydroxyvitamin D concentrations, and safety." The American Journal of Clinical Nutrition; May 1999:69(5)842-856.

[15] Hathcock, JN. Et al, "Risk assessment of vitamin D." The American Journal of Clinical Nutrition; January 2007:84(1) 5-18.

[16] Haddad, JG. et al, "Human plasma transport of vitamin D after its endogenous synthesis." Journal of Clinical Investigation; 1993:91(6)2552-2555.

[17] Ross, AC. et al., "The 2011 report on dietary reference intakes for calcium and vitamin D from the Institute of Medicine, what clinicians need to know." J. Clin. Endocrinol. Metab.; January 2011:96(1) 53-58.

[18] Vitamin D; Merck Manual of Diagnosis and Therapy, Professional Edition.

[19] Tuohimaa, P., "Vitamin D and aging." The Journal of Steroid Biochemistry and Molecular Biology; March 2009: 114(1-2) 78-84.

[20] Ansell, J. et al., "The pharmacology and management of the vitamin K antagonists:the Seventh ACCP Conference on Antithrombotic and Thrombolytic Therapy." Chest, 2004; 126(3 Suppl):204-233.

[21] Groenen-van Dooren, MM.,"Bioavailability of phylloquinone and menaquinones after oral and colorectal administration in vitamin K deficient rats." Biochem Pharmacol, Sept 7, 1995;50(6):797-801.

[22] Binkley N et al,"A high phylloquinone intake is required to achieve maximal osteocalcin (gamma)-carboxylation."American Journal of Clinical Nutrition, 76(5).

[23] Colditz, G, "Selenium and Cancer Prevention." JAMA,1996; 276(24):1984-1985.

[24] Yang, C., "Research on Esophageal Cancer in China: a Review." Cancer Research, 1980;40:2633.

[25] Schroder, J, "Discovery of resveratrol." Resveratrol; March 6, 2010.

[26] Howitz, KT, et al., "Small molecule activators of sirtuins extend Sacchomyces cerevisiae lifespan." Nature, Sept. 2003;425(6954): 191-196.

[27] Kuskoski EM, et al, "Wild fruits and pulps of frozen fruits:antioxidant activity, polyphenols and proanthrocyins"

[28] Schauss AG et al, "Antioxidant capacity and other bioactivities of the freeze-dried amazonian palm berry, Euterpe oleraceae Mart. (acai)." J Agri Food Chem;54(22) 8504-8610.

[29] Ovivnikov, A.M., "A theory of marginotomy. The incomplete copying of template margin in enzymatic synthesis of polynucleotides and biological significance of the phenomenon." J. Theor. Biol.,Sept. 1973;41(1):181-190.

[30] Blasko, M.A., "Telomeres and disease: aging, cancer and beyond." Nat. Rev. Genet.,Aug 2005;6(8):611-622.

[31] Shay, J.W. & Bacchetti, S., "A survey of telomerase activity in human cancer." Eur. J. Cancer, Apr 1997;33(5):787-791.

8

EXERCISE AND HEALTH

As I alluded to in the chapter in which I defined anti-aging medicine, exercise is a very important part of an overall program. For those who are unaccustomed to any type of exercise, it is recommended to start a program slowly and deliberately. Walking to the mailbox is enough for people who have been sedentary for years. That simple activity puts a person in the frame of mind of doing something active, regardless of the level. When that same person gets accustomed to walking to the mailbox daily, then the natural tendency is to do more, and that could result in walking past the mailbox for increasing distances. Ultimately, that will result in a walking program that will actually benefit the person by increasing their activity level, thereby increasing their metabolic demand and capacity. A secondary goal for a walking program can be walking a total of thirty uninterrupted minutes a day. That alone will be successful in improving that person's overall health.

Another excellent form of exercise is swimming, but obviously, one has to have access to a pool. In comparison to walking, swimming incorporates many other muscles, and places a higher metabolic demand on the body. When metabolic demand increases, the human body accommodates gradually to meet that demand by increasing the capacity to tolerate the activity. That's called getting into shape or conditioning! It is always wise to talk to a trusted doctor before beginning any exercise routine.

If one wants to optimize an exercise program and increase strength and muscle mass, then progressive resistive exercise

(PRE) has been shown to accomplish that goal. Research has shown that the very best way to perform PRE is by using dumbbells or kettle bells. The reason is because one must control the weight in space as well as lifting the poundage. It is easier to control a barbell as opposed to a dumbbell because each dumbbell is held in one hand, while using a barbell requires the simultaneous use of both hands. Using a machine, regardless of the make or model, does not require controlling the weight in space and as a result, the machines are not quite as effective, but are easier to use. The advantage of a machine is being able to combine all exercises with the use of one machine (universal) in some cases. If one is unable to gain access to dumbbells, using a machine or barbells are certainly okay, but not optimal. Every weight training program is different and should be changed to meet an individual's needs on a periodic basis. The longer one sticks with a program, the more times they will change the various exercises in order to meet their needs.

One should not ignore the issue of hydration which is even more important with an exercise program. It is important to remain hydrated by drinking water particularly if the ambient temperature is elevated or if one is over the age of sixty-five.[1] The urine of a properly hydrated person is relatively clear while a darker yellow color is consistent with dehydration.[2]

A basic program includes general exercises for all body parts and the program should not last more than forty-five minutes. I recommend using a comfortable weight for each exercise that one can perform at least eight to twelve times. Performing the same exercise through one range of motion is called a repetition, and when eight to twelve repetitions are performed, that is referred to as a "set." In the beginning stages, I recommend performing only one set of each particular exercise and continue with the one set routine for the first two to three weeks. This allows one to get used to the exercises and learn how the exercises are to be performed without the chance of injury. Only after a person is comfortable with each exercise and has gained an improvement in their strength should they attempt to increase the number of sets to two. The length of time that one waits between performing one set and the next set will depend upon the degree of fitness. If those exercising find themselves having trouble catching their breath or becoming fatigued, then they must wait longer between sets. If one experiences chest pain, shortness of breath, pain or numbness in their left arm or neck, then he/she should stop the program and consider undergoing a stress test to determine whether or not there is any type of heart problem. If one is not feeling pain, numbness or shortness of breath, but simply feeling tired, then it is most likely a conditioning issue. The conditioning issue will gradually resolve and the time between sets will shorten as a result. Highly trained athletes may only wait thirty to forty-five seconds between sets, so if a person finds only a minute or so is needed between sets, then the conditioning is actually very good. Remember that the person exercising is not competing with anyone else, nor should that person compare with others around them. People should always exercise at their own pace and only compare themselves with themselves at previous point in time. That is the reason why one should make out a chart of exercises with the poundage used, along with the number of repetitions and sets. People should make certain to record the date so that they can compare themselves to what they were doing a month, six months, or a year earlier. It will pleasantly surprise most people when they see their progress, not to mention the change in their body shape.

Once a person has decided to engage in a PRE program, then he or she must determine the specific exercises to incorporate. For the novice, I recommend a basic program that includes exercises for the largest muscle groups first. For example, the quadriceps mechanism in the thigh is a large muscle group, and the hamstrings are as well. The chest and back are also considered large muscle groups. The quadriceps (quads) are named that because there are actually four (4) muscles in the quads, the vastus medialis, vastus intermedius, vastus lateralis and the rectus femoris. The function of the quadriceps is to straighten the knee and hold the lower extremity straight. For the quads, I recommend grasping a dumbbell in each hand and placing the feet at shoulder width. Then, perform a deep knee bend (squat) as far as you can, but stop at a point when the thighs are parallel to the floor. If you are not able to go that far, that's fine, but go as far as you can without pain or discomfort. Perform that exercise eight to twelve times and use a weight that is comfortable, but a degree of difficulty should be noted with the last 1 or 2 repetitions. Wait about two minutes before moving to the next set. If you need more time, that's okay because remember I said that the person should go at one's own pace.

The next set should involve the hamstrings which are the large muscles in the back of the thigh that are responsible for bending the knee. For this particular muscle group, one needs either weighted boots or a leg curl machine. The weighted boots will allow the person to exercise each thigh individually, but if these are not available, then a leg curl machine is the only answer. Again, perform eight to twelve repetitions using a weight that is comfortable. One should be able to perform the exercise without "jerking" the weight, so start with low poundage. Wait for a comfortable time interval and then move on to the next exercise for another "large" muscle group.

I recommend an exercise for the back muscles next which involves mostly the latissimus dorsi muscle. Exercise one side at a time, but both sides can be done simultaneously. It's easier to do one side at a time because one can balance with the other side. Holding the dumbbell in one hand, bend forward at the waist to about 80 or 90 degrees. Use the other unoccupied hand for balance, and while in the bent forward position, allow the arm holding the weight to simply hang straight down. The arm will be straight and perpendicular to the floor at that point and the palm will be closest to the body. The exercise is called "rowing" and it consists of raising the weight (dumbbell) upward until it touches one's side just below their chest. Perform eight to twelve repetitions and then rest. If you find yourself straining excessively or jerking in order to perform the movement, then you need to reduce the poundage. Again, rest for the period of time you need before the next exercise set.

The chest muscles should be next as they are also considered a large muscle group. For the next exercise, one will need a bench that is approximately ten to twelve inches in width. Bench widths vary, but the main thing to remember is that it should be comfortable and allow you to move your arms in an unimpeded manner. The dumbbells are placed in the hands while you sit on the end of the bench. The dumbbells are raised to the shoulders by bending the arms and then lie down on the bench with your head at one end and your bottom at the other. When you have assumed the reclining position on your back, the dumbbells are rotated so that the palms face inward toward the body. One can also perform this exercise on the floor, but it is easier to use a bench. Begin with the dumbbells close to the sides in the chest area, but do not lower the dumbbells to a point where the arms go beyond being parallel to the floor. Then straighten the arms until the weights are above the chest, with the elbows straightened, perpendicular to the bench or floor. When raising the dumbbells, the hands are rotated so that the palms are facing the feet when the elbows are straight. The reason the rotation is done is to reduce stress on the shoulders. When the dumbbells are lowered, rotate the hands back to the original position, remembering not to lower them any lower than when the arm (shoulder to elbow) is parallel with the floor. Perform the same exercise eight to twelve times (repetitions). Rest after the last repetition before the next set which will be for the triceps, or the muscles that straighten the arm.

One may use the floor for the triceps exercise, but a bench is preferred. While lying on the back and holding the dumbbell by the side of the head with the palms facing the head, simply straighten the elbow which will result in raising the weight above and slightly to the side of the head. One may perform this exercise with each hand individually or both hands simultaneously for eight to twelve repetitions. Again, rest for the regular rest time before the next exercise (arm curls) that will be for the arm flexors.

Curls are performed by grasping the dumbbells in each hand while standing or sitting. With the palms facing forward and stabilizing the elbows by one's side, bend the elbows which will result in raising the weights toward the shoulders. After bending the elbows as much as possible, the weights are then returned to the starting position slowly and subsequently repeated until eight to twelve repetitions are completed. Rest again before starting the next exercise for the shoulders.

While holding a dumbbell in each hand by the sides, raise the dumbbells out from each side with the thumbs pointing upward. Perform eight to twelve slow repetitions and then perform another set, but this time raise the dumbbells to the front, again with the thumbs pointing upward. Rest at that point in order to get ready for the next to the last exercise.

The next exercise is designed to strengthen the calves. With dumbbells in each hand by the sides, rise onto the balls of the feet until you can rise no higher. This exercise is best performed using a one to two inch block under the balls of the feet. This allows additional range of motion for the ankles and will result in the development of stronger and larger calves. Rest again and then perform eight to twelve bent knee sit-ups on the floor or a bench. If possible, another person can assist in stabilizing the feet, as it prevents someone from using motion with the legs to assist with a sit-up. Do not jerk while performing this exercise and do not pull on the back of the head in an attempt to help with the motion. This exercise is designed to strengthen the abdominal muscles, so one should avoid using other muscles to assist. If one is unable to perform eight to twelve repetitions, don't worry; simply perform the maximum number of comfortable repetitions and things will improve.

The biggest problem I have witnessed with exercise programs is that many see exercise as a negative task instead of enjoyment. That happens when the person tries to do too much by attempting to keep up with others. By doing too much, exercise does become a chore, plus one stands the chance of being injured and that defeats the whole purpose of exercise. The other factor to keep in mind is the duration of an exercise routine. I have advised athletes, both amateur and professional, for a number of years about the time limit for an exercise routine. Many people (most athletes) over-train and that can result in a negative experience by making it a chore or causing injuries. Keep it simple and short as an exercise program routine should never go beyond forty-five minutes. Avoid over-training as the potential problems far outweigh the benefits and will jeopardize attempts to optimize one's health. It is recommended that the above PRE exercise program should be performed at least three to four times per week. Also, when performing exercise with resistance (PRE), many people forget to breathe. Unbelievable as that sounds, many people hold their breath during PRE until the set is concluded or they breathe erratically. When performing a concentric contraction (the muscle that is being exercised is contracting), one should inhale. When the weight is returned to the original position, the person should exhale.[3] All movements should be purposeful and deliberate and should never be done rapidly or with a jerking motion.

For those who become interested in advanced PRE training, a split routine can be incorporated, whereby only individual muscle groups are trained every three days. For example, one day can consist of training only the chest, triceps, and shoulders. By the time a person considers a split routine, they will have advanced to the point of performing three sets of each exercise in a basic total body program as referred to earlier. Accordingly, each individual exercise for a given body area should include at least three sets. In this example, a person would perform three sets of dumbbell bench presses of eight to ten repetitions each. Additional exercises can be added to individual body areas. In the case of the chest, supine lateral raises could be added. This exercise is best performed on a bench. The person lies on his/her back with a dumbbell in each hand with the palms up and the elbows bent to about thirty to forty-five degrees. Starting with the weights by the side (similar to the bench press), the weights are lowered to the side until the arms are basically parallel to the floor. At that point, the weights are raised upward until they meet midline above the upper chest. Repeat the same maneuver eight to ten times for a total of three sets. In all cases, when a person has never performed that particular exercise before, it is best to start with one set and gradually increase as tolerated. With this exercise, as with bench presses, be cautious to not allow the arms to go too far to the floor because it could result in injury to the shoulders, especially in those not accustomed to those exercises. Once the sets for the chest are completed, it is advisable to work the shoulders the same way as noted in the basic overall workout routine. The only addition is an exercise for the posterior aspect of the rotator cuff that is done by holding the dumbbells in both hands by the sides while bending forward at the waist to about forty-five degrees. While in that position, raise the weights upward and backward while keeping the elbows slightly bent. In most cases, the arms (that portion of the upper extremity beginning at the shoulder and ending at the elbow) will be parallel with the floor at the end of that lift. Let the weights return to the sides and repeat eight to ten times. As indicated, the total shoulder program will also include raising the dumbbells to the side and front for eight to ten repetitions as well. It is recommended that most people begin with minimum weight, as those muscles are usually weak because they are rarely exercised. It surprises most people when they discover the minimal amount of weight necessary to provide sufficient resistance. Remember not to use too little weight, but on the other hand, don't use too much as it defeats the purpose of isolating the muscle groups to be exercised. It is not unusual to use two to three pound dumbbells in each hand when starting the exercise program for the shoulders. Each person is different and will have different capabilities. Use a comfortable poundage that will allow the performance of each exercise without jerking or throwing. The last repetition should always be somewhat more strenuous than the others, and if not, the poundage is too little. The next exercise on day one will be for the triceps, or the muscle group that extends the forearm and straightens the elbow. Lie on your back and grasp one dumbbell with both hands or use a dumbbell in each hand. The weights are placed next to the head and grasped with the thumbs pointing toward the floor. The weight or weights are then raised above the head until the arms are straight and then allowed to return to the position by the head. The same maneuver is repeated for eight to ten repetitions for three sets. That concludes the first day using a split routine.

For years, exercise has been divided between aerobic and anaerobic. PRE is referred to as being anaerobic; however, if the person allows only minimal periods of rest between sets, then PRE can become aerobic exercise as well. For example, a person who waits two to three minutes between sets will not build their aerobic capacity because the rest allows the respiration and heart beat to return to baseline. In order to get a simultaneous aerobic workout with PRE, the rest periods can be no longer than thirty seconds and can certainly be less depending on the level of conditioning. In the beginning stages, it is advisable to approach this time limit gradually and only to tolerance. Once a person is able to rest thirty seconds or less between sets, he/she is also engaging in aerobic exercise. Of course, if one prefers, a separate aerobic exercise program can be utilized.

The second day of a split routine exercise program will feature a separate group of muscles including the back, biceps, and abdominal muscles. For the back, it is suggested to perform the previously described rowing motion that is done while bent forward at the waist while providing support with the free hand. Again, perform eight to ten repetitions for at least three sets. There are variations to this exercise and entire books are available on the subject for the interested and motivated person. The next exercise is bent knee sit-ups as described in the general program. It is advisable to begin with at least three sets of fifteen repetitions. If others are available, it helps if they stabilize the person's feet during this exercise by either holding the feet against the floor with their hands or sitting on the feet. The hands are not held behind the head, they simply touch the head on either side. That prevents the person from using arm strength to pull the head up and forward. The exercise is designed to strengthen the abdominal muscles only. The next and last exercise for day two of the split routine is for the flexors of the arm. This is accomplished by performing the curls described previously.

The third day is devoted to the lower extremities, wherein the workout will include exercise for the knee extensors (quadriceps), knee flexors (hamstrings), and calves. Those exercises were previously described. Each muscle group should be exercised for ten to twelve repetitions for three sets.

At that point, one starts the program again on the fourth day. Day seven is a rest day and the process begins again on the eighth day. Keep in mind that there are many exercises available for the same muscle groups. The recommendations I have offered simply provide a starting point and one may add or subtract various exercises as long as it helps achieve a goal. There are numerous exercise instruction books readily available at bookstores and libraries for the person wishing to fine tune and train at a higher level.

Aerobic exercise is defined as that type of exercise that uses oxygen to generate energy, and can be performed in a variety of ways. As I indicated with PRE, not only is it considered anaerobic, but it can be aerobic as well. However, purists refer to such things as jogging, swimming, long distance running, stair climbing, elliptical training, cycling, rowing, cross-country skiing, inline skating, kickboxing, jumping rope, and Nordic walking as being aerobic exercise. Generally speaking, aerobic exercise is performed at a moderate level of intensity over a relatively long period of time. Aerobic exercise helps strengthen muscles of breathing and the heart. It can also help strengthen other muscles of the body depending upon the exercise undertaken. It can help improve blood pressure and circulatory efficiency and it can help reduce the risk for type II diabetes. Because of the attendant reduction of stress seen with aerobic exercise, it can also help with depression. Aerobic exercise of some type can be performed prior to or after a PRE program if the PRE program includes excessive wait times between sets. Most experts agree that an aerobic exercise program should be performed a minimum of three times per week for a minimum of twenty minutes each time.

Please keep in mind that the foregoing is a guide for those who desire to change their metabolic status and overall health by improving their strength, endurance, and metabolic capacity. Without some type of regular exercise, one can't achieve optimum health.

As with many other aspects of achieving optimal health, there are a number of myths associated with exercise. Some people feel as though they are too old to exercise, but that is typically an excuse and not a valid reason for those who have managed to maintain a healthy status. That healthy status is dependent on a number of other factors, including metabolic optimization as a result of appropriate supplementation with hormones and a proper dietary regimen. Once those parameters are met, the next health optimizing benefit is derived from a regular exercise program of some sort. Another excuse is the lack of time, but again, that's an excuse not a reason. Everyone has the time, but everyone doesn't have their time prioritized properly in regard to optimizing their health. A number of female patients have told me that they didn't want to look like a man so they didn't want to engage in PRE. It is a myth that women will develop a physique similar to men, because that phenomenon will occur only if their hormone balance is improper. In other words, if a woman has an inappropriately high level of testosterone, then PRE can cause muscular growth similar to that seen in a male. However, that is atypical and simply doesn't happen in most females. Because of the above noted misconception, many women will only engage in aerobic exercise. Of course, some form of exercise is better than no exercise, but avoiding PRE is a mistake and only allows the person partial benefit. When working out, discard the military motto of "no pain, no gain." It doesn't work and should never be a part of any exercise program. If one experiences pain with any exercise, something is wrong! If it is the result of soreness during the initial phases of an exercise program, then it will resolve after the first two weeks or so. However, pain complaints after that time are not normal and should be dealt with in a logical manner, and that does not include continuing the same exercise that hurts. Regardless of what exercise gurus and physical therapy experts may claim, one will exacerbate an underlying soft tissue injury or condition with exercise and should not continue to perform an exercise of an injured body part. If one incorporates a new exercise in their program, they should expect some temporary soreness that will resolve as noted above.

Other benefits from a regular exercise program include sustained fat loss as the result of increasing the basal metabolic rate due to increasing the lean body mass (muscle tissue.) Muscle tissue has a higher metabolic demand than fat and a higher metabolic demand results in the necessity of getting that extra fuel from either the diet or stored body fuel in the form of glycogen or fat. In turn, that can result in the use of stored fat as an energy source, and that is further manifested by fat weight loss with a change in the body shape. In addition, engaging in exercise results in the release of endorphins and the neurotransmitters dopamine, serotonin, and norepinephrine. Elevation of those substances is effective in improving the mood and counteracting depression.

Notes

[1] "Exercise and Fluid Replacement." American College of Sports Medicine.

[2] Johnson-Cane D. et al, *The Complete Idiot's Guide to Weight Training*, 2000; Indianapolis, Alpha Books: 169.

[3] Ibid.,152.

9

PROLOTHERAPY/RIT

I would be remiss to not include a chapter on this fascinating but relatively unknown treatment method. In the preface of this book, I discussed how a board certified specialist in Physical Medicine and Rehabilitation became interested in hormone replacement and other factors that enhance health and healing. The orthopedic surgeon had been treated by me previously with prolotherapy (prolo), aka regenerative injection therapy (RIT) or sclerotherapy, hereafter abbreviated as RIT, for a problem with his knee. This particular orthopedic surgeon was also an avid golfer who considered the golf course his "zen" place. He sought the help of his orthopedic surgeon colleagues, and after several weeks of injections and exercise, his knee pain had not improved. The more important fact to understand is that he had not been able to play golf. He had heard of RIT, but since it was the general consensus of his orthopedic colleagues that it did not work, he deferred looking into it further. As a last resort, he called me and asked if I would mind taking a look at his problem knee. After reviewing imaging studies and examining him, I told him that he had an enthesitis (inflammation of the attachments) of the medial collateral ligament and the medial portion of the quadriceps tendon. That means that he had sustained microscopic tearing of the medial collateral ligament fibers that attach to the femur (thigh bone) on one end and the tibia (leg bone) on the other end. A similar thing had also occurred to the quadriceps tendon at its attachment to the patella (knee cap). An enthesis is simply the site where a tendon, ligament, or capsule attaches to bone. When microscopic tearing like that occurs, exercise is not helpful; to the contrary, exercise typically makes it worse. Of course, his colleagues prescribed an exercise program for him after injecting a steroid into his knee joint. Not only did they fail to inject the correct structures, but they also made his problem worse with exercise. I explained the situation to him and he agreed to undergo RIT even though he had been told it "didn't work." I injected his knee in three locations with an RIT solution and asked him to return to my office after two weeks. Upon his return, he indicated that his pain was almost gone and that he had visited the golf driving range to see if he could tolerate a golf swing. To his amazement, the swing was virtually pain-free, but a slight degree of pain remained that I was able to resolve with a second series of injections. Needless to say, he became a fan of RIT, and subsequently referred the patient I spoke of in the preface that started my quest in regard to hormone replacement.

I became aware of RIT in 1977 during my internship in Phoenix, Arizona. A fellow doctor in training was a jogger and told me that he was going to try RIT in order to treat a tendonitis of his heel. We discussed it and I asked a number of questions since I'd never heard of such a treatment before. To my surprise, the treatment was to be done by one of the doctors in the Physical Medicine and Rehabilitation (PM&R) department. Since I was to start training in that field after my internship, my interest was genuine. I was able to meet Dr. Kent Pomeroy who introduced me to RIT.

When most people hear about injecting a joint, a tendon or a ligament, they automatically assume that the structure will be injected with a corticosteroid (cortisone). Most doctors have that same impression as well, and prior to hearing and learning about RIT, I was just as naïve as everyone else. RIT uses different solutions, but none are similar or even remotely related to cortisone. The difference is significant and the results are different as well. Cortisone is an anti-inflammatory drug that suppresses cellular activity, reduces swelling, and results in pain relief as a result of blocking pain-producing substances. **Unfortunately, cortisone does not promote healing; to the contrary, it makes the injected tissues weaker and more prone to further injury**. RIT works by strengthening tissues as a result of stimulating the release of specific growth factors for those tissues. In the case of tendons, it works by stimulating release of growth factors that stimulate growth of new tendon tissue. The same phenomenon works for ligaments and the capsules surrounding all joints.

RIT is essentially the opposite of injecting a tissue with a corticosteroid, aka cortisone (anti-inflammatory). As indicated above, cortisone does not promote healing; to the contrary, it actually weakens the tissue injected. RIT works by stimulating the healing response at the injection site which is always next to the attachment site (enthesis) of ligaments, tendons, and capsules with bone. Healing is divided into three phases: inflammatory, proliferative, and remodeling. The inflammatory phase begins when a RIT solution is injected at an enthesis. **The inflammatory phase lasts from one to three days** and begins when the injected solution causes the cells at that site to rupture and release their contents into the surrounding area. Many substances within the contents are chemically active and trigger an inflammatory response that starts the cascade of healing. Growth factors are also released that stimulate the influx of cells that manufacture new native collagen and elastin cells. Collagen and elastin are the primary constituents of ligament, tendon, and capsular tissues. White blood cells are attracted to the site as well, and other cells, known as macrophages, act to "clean up" the site by removing needless cellular debris. **Next is the proliferative phase that lasts ten to fourteen days.** During that phase, other cells are attracted to the site by cellular growth factors and induce further healing. One particular type of cell, known as a "fibroblast," is instrumental in the deposition of new native collagen and elastin tissue. New blood vessels are also stimulated to form in the newly developing tissue, in order to ensure that the cells get enough oxygen. **The last phase is the remodeling phase and can last up to one year.** During that time, the new tissue matures and strengthens as the collagen forms according to the function it is to assume. In other words, if it is the job of a ligament to resist force in a certain direction, then the ligament will develop in that manner and stabilize the structures for movement in that direction. During the proliferative and remodeling phases, it is important for the patient to perform normal range of motion movements that stimulate the developing tissues to grow in the proper direction, so as to provide proper support and stabilization.

Most patients require from three to six visits, at two to three week intervals, in order to facilitate maximum healing. Each time a patient undergoes an RIT injection, the previously described three phases are again stimulated to take place. It is not unusual for patients to achieve total relief of their symptoms of pain and/or weakness once treatment is completed. The injected tissue can actually become stronger than before the area was injured.

Some ask what the rationale for recommending RIT might be. Tissues like ligaments, tendons, and joint capsules have a very poor blood supply at their attachment site to bone. A reduced blood supply results in a poor oxygen and nutrient supply, resulting in impaired healing. Younger people possess a higher probability of healing typically because the blood supply is better, and there is usually no metabolic imbalance because hormones are at their peak in younger individuals. RIT typically works quite well in younger individuals because of those reasons. However, as a person ages, the supply of blood to attachment sites gradually decreases and hormones characteristically decline as well. Young people can typically undergo RIT for healing without having to analyze their hormonal status. On the other hand, the one factor that reduces the effectiveness in older individuals is hormonal balance. For that reason, it is wise to check hormonal levels prior to undergoing RIT for patients over forty.

If a ligament, tendon, or capsule is going to heal on its own, the majority of healing will take place within five to six weeks. Pain is commonly the presenting symptom when those tissues are injured, and if the pain does not resolve, the tissue has not healed. When the pain continues after five to six weeks, it is time to consider local measures, such as ice massage and ultrasound treatment, provided the patient's hormonal status is optimal. Those modalities can also be used prior to that time as well simply to speed the healing process. If the pain persists at the same or higher level after four additional weeks, then RIT should be considered as a treatment option. RIT is also appropriate for loose ligaments, hypermobile joints, unstable joints, joint space narrowing, chronic sprains, or with conditions that temporarily improve with mobilization and manipulation treatment.

How does one know whether or not they have a condition that might improve with RIT? The doctor must first perform a proper physical examination before ordering imaging studies such as MRIs, CAT scans, and x-rays. Within that exam, the doctor should pay strict attention to any finding suggesting involvement of the neurological system. The reason is that a small percentage of patients may have compromise of the nerves exiting the spine (nerve roots) that could possibly be helped with surgery. If compromise of a nerve root is suspected, the patient should undergo electrodiagnostic studies that will be discussed later. Most patients have no abnormal neurological findings, but even then, the doctor may place far too much emphasis on imaging studies without ever touching the patient. Conditions that may respond to RIT are those with pain that is typically worse when remaining in any one position for an extended time, such as with standing or sitting. There is usually consistent specific tenderness to pressure over the area involved, and if the tendon, ligament, or joint capsule is injected with a local anesthetic such as lidocaine, the pain is relieved temporarily, either partially or completely. When pain is relieved in this manner, range of motion is typically restored as well. RIT is not indicated for injuries that are acute because the patient's natural healing process might result in optimal healing. As noted before, if pain does not improve gradually with the passage of time as noted above and the use of local treatment with ice massage and/or ultrasound, then RIT should be considered.

The term prolotherapy is derived from the Latin word "proles" that means growth or offspring. Regardless of the term used, the philosophy of using this particular treatment method is rooted in antiquity, as Hippocrates was known to cauterize injured shoulder joint capsules for stabilization. Cauterization was used for centuries to stop bleeding and coalesce tissues. Beginning in the 1930s, surgeons used various injected solutions to help heal hernias and hydroceles. The first tissue study about the results of RIT was performed in the 1930s as well. Dr. Porritt treated bursitis of the elbow and knee with RIT using a solution known as sodium morrhuate.[1] Dr. Louis Shultz injected temporomandibular joint capsules (TMJ) with proliferants and recommended injecting other joint capsules as well.[2] In 1937, Dr. Earl Gedney reported injecting spinal discs and sprained ligaments with proliferant solutions.

In 1938, Drs. Steindler and Luck postulated that there was a great deal of confusion between structural and neural components in the lumbosacral spine (lower back). Similar levels of pain can result from an injury to a nerve or a tissue like a ligament, tendon, or joint capsule. Pain can radiate in a similar pattern from the injury sites as well. It is the task of a true science-minded physician to know the difference. This ongoing confusion has led to untold numbers of patients undergoing needless spinal surgery and has led to the diagnosis of "failed back syndrome." In 1938, doctors injected local anesthetic into sacroiliac joints that stopped complaints of lower back pain in those patients. That led to the conclusion that SI joint dysfunction was one of the definite causes of lower back pain that could be confused with nerve root pain.[3] **That was over seventy years ago and the same confusion persists today!**

In 1939, a young surgeon, Dr. George Hackett from Canton, Ohio, began researching ligament pain. Dr. Hackett postulated that most lower back pain was the result of "ligament relaxation," and in 1956, he introduced the term prolotherapy. In the same year, Dr. Hackett published his research regarding pain referral patterns from ligaments and tendons. Dr. Hackett also recognized that pain also emanated from tendons and referred to that phenomenon as "tendon relaxation." We now know and understand that the ligaments and tendons are not relaxed; the pain actually originates at the site where the tendon or ligament attach to bone and is caused by microscopic tearing.

In the late 1960s, a patient died as the result of RIT and another patient was paralyzed. After researching the issue, it became apparent that the procedures were performed by unqualified and inexperienced physicians. It is very rare for patients to experience any serious side effects with RIT performed by a knowledgeable and skilled physician.

In 1963 a significant study was published showing a seventy-five percent cure rate for traumatic headaches treated with RIT. During the following years, a number of studies showed the tremendous benefit of RIT in treating ligaments, tendons, and capsules at their attachment sites. It is important to understand that this type of pain originates at the site where the tissue attaches to bone.

We know without question that RIT is quite effective in treating injured tissues such as ligaments, tendons, and joint capsules. I have used this treatment method for over thirty years and have found it to offer tremendous benefit for many previously undiagnosed or improperly diagnosed conditions. Many patients have been surprised that other doctors had not suggested such a viable treatment prior to coming to my clinic. A number of those same patients had been forced to live with unrelenting pain simply because doctors are not educated about the subject of RIT.

Throughout my career, I have seen literally thousands of patients with complaints of lower back pain. Most had seen their family doctor, orthopedist, neurologist, and/or neurosurgeon. If they had back pain for more than few weeks, most had undergone an MRI. If an MRI showed a herniated disc, then that patient may have ended up under the surgeon's knife without any further studies. Unfortunately, there are false positive MRIs that appear to show abnormalities that aren't really there at the time of surgery. What most people don't understand is that an MRI is simply an imaging (photographic) study that shows anatomy. It does not show anything about function. A person without back pain may have an MRI that coincidentally shows a herniated disc. Does that mean they need surgery? Absolutely not! Finding a herniated or bulging disc does not mean a person has pain or needs surgery. If that's the case, why operate on someone simply based upon the result of an MRI study? The answer to that dilemma is to undergo a careful and thorough physical examination. If there are true neurological findings such as loss of strength, abnormal reflexes, and sensory abnormalities, then surgery might be considered as necessary. However, before surgery is considered, then the patient should absolutely and unequivocally undergo electrodiagnostic testing (EMGs and/or nerve conduction studies). Those studies, as compared to MRIs, determine physiology (function of the living organism). In other words, the studies help determine if the anatomical abnormality such as a ruptured (herniated) disc is actually causing a problem with any of the nerves. If the physical examination reveals neurological abnormalities, the MRI shows an abnormality that corresponds to the examination findings, and the EMG is abnormal, surgery is a viable course to pursue if the patient is not showing signs of improvement. Surgery is not a course to pursue without those findings because once surgery is performed, it can't be reversed.

Up to ninety-percent of lower back pain is generated from ligaments, tendons, and/or joint capsules. When those structures degenerate with age or are injured, microscopic tearing can and often does occur at the point where they attach and anchor to bone. That is referred to as the fibro-osseous junction or the enthesis. In order for those structures to attach, fibers from those tissues actually penetrate the bone in order to provide maximum stability. At every attachment site are literally tens of thousands, if not millions, of fibers. It takes only a small percentage of those fibers to tear in order to cause pain. The bone is covered with a layer of tissue called the periosteum (surrounding bone) that has a rich network of pain sensitive nerves called C-fibers. C-fibers only do one thing; **they transmit pain messages** to the brain if and when they are stimulated. If a patient fractures a bone, it results in the disruption and stimulation of those C-fibers and the patient perceives that as pain. The fibers that result in the pain of a fracture are the same fibers that are activated when microscopic tearing of ligaments, tendons, or joint capsules occur at the enthesis.

Microscopic tearing cannot be identified by an x-ray, MRI, or EMG. In order to make the diagnosis, the doctor must be able to examine the patient properly and interpret the findings. The majority of doctors are not trained to find these common problems even though it is responsible for most lower back pain. I will also mention again, it is what your doctor doesn't know that can hurt you.

The following is the typical story that I get from patients who have lower back pain that has been present more than three or four months. Most either visited an emergency room with the onset of symptoms or saw their family doctor. They were prescribed pain medication along with some type of NSAID (non-steroidal anti-inflammatory drug) and a muscle relaxer type of drug. By the way, muscle relaxers don't really relax muscles directly, they simply cause sedation. For those who are healthy and have a good healing response, their pain subsides and I never hear from them unless they aggravate their underlying problem later. For those who have persisting pain, their family doctor typically refers them to an orthopedic surgeon who most people consider to be the "expert" on lower back pain. Please keep in mind that half their specialty title is "surgeon." Also, be mindful of the fact that I'm simply repeating the story I have heard countless times and this is not meant to be a condescending inference about orthopedic surgeons. Once the patient goes to the orthopedist, they are immediately x-rayed in order to determine whether or not there is a skeletal problem such as a fracture, arthritic change, or disc narrowing. If none of those problems are identified, the patient is typically instructed to undergo an MRI. If there is any suggestion of disc disease, that patient may end up in a surgical suite undergoing inappropriate surgery. That is certainly not true of most orthopedic surgeons, but I have seen a number of horror stories in that regard. If the MRI shows no problem, then the patient is given a prescription for physical therapy that usually reads something like, "evaluate and treat." Any prescription written in that manner simply shows that the doctor writing the prescription doesn't have a clue. It would be similar to a prescription just saying, "provide drugs to this patient." The patient may be told that they don't have a surgical problem and to expect improvement on a gradual basis with physical therapy. They may or may not be given a prescription for pain medication, muscle relaxers, and anti-inflammatory medication. The problem with that common scenario is that the typical orthopedist doesn't know the cause of the patient's pain and provides a general diagnosis of a lumbosacral sprain or non-discogenic lower back pain. What does that mean? Again, it means the orthopedist has no clue about the cause of the persisting pain. Nevertheless, the patient is sent to an equally uninformed physical therapist (PT) upon whom is placed the burden of getting the patient better. In other words, for all intents and purposes, the orthopedist hands off patient responsibility to the PT. Many PTs have no clue in regard to what causes ninety-percent of lower back pain either and treat virtually everyone with exercise. Ask yourself a logical question and one that seems to never be considered by orthopedists, neurologists, neurosurgeons, family doctors, or PTs. How does a torn tissue heal if someone keeps pulling and stressing it with exercise? In the case of torn ligaments, tendons, and joint capsules, it does not benefit them at all. To the contrary, it typically makes things worse by causing more injury and preventing healing. Unfortunately for the patient, this leads many PTs to assume that the patient is not performing the exercises properly or the patient has no motivation to improve. How utterly silly is that? The logical thought process would have most individuals think that exercise might be causing the problem to worsen, but because of incorrect training, many PTs and equally uninformed doctors continue to push exercise. When the patient returns to the orthopedist or other doctor still complaining of pain in spite of an exercise program, they are looked at as complainers or people with ulterior motives. Instead of the doctors questioning their diagnosis and treatment program, they blame the failure on the patient. I've always found that very disconcerting.

Instead of the above described situation, involving a patient with non-surgical lower back pain, orthopedic surgeons in particular and other doctors in general should make a concerted effort to learn how to diagnose the major causes of lower back pain. The other alternative is to refer the patient to a knowledgeable doctor who is trained properly and knows how to make those diagnoses. Instead of relying upon imaging studies that will not reveal anything about microscopic tearing, the examining doctor must understand the anatomical structures and pathophysiology involved that cause most lower back pain. Unless the doctor knows those things, he/she will miss the majority of causes of lower back pain. By knowing the anatomical structures and the proper method of examining the patient, the doctor understands how to arrive at the proper diagnosis. The doctor **must touch** the patient in order to elicit the typical findings. I will guarantee that many reading this book have been to a doctor because of lower back pain. It would not be surprising to me that many of those patients were never touched by the examining physician. It is virtually impossible to identify and diagnose ligament, tendon, or joint capsular problems without touching the patient! Palpation (applying varying degrees of pressure with the hands) to affected structures is a must! Without a proper diagnosis, is it logical or even probable that the doctor will prescribe treatment that will benefit the patient? Obviously not, and that's one of the reasons why millions of people have to deal with back pain on a daily basis. If this sounds logical and rational, it's because it is! So why is the standard of care so substandard and limited in regard to treating most conditions involving lower back pain? It goes back to what I have indicated before about training programs being inadequate. When microscopic tearing occurs, the area becomes painful and very sensitive to the touch because a number of pain producing substances are released when the area is injured. When those areas are palpated, the affected areas will become quite evident because of the amount of pain produced. If that step is omitted from an examination, one can begin to see why those doctors miss the diagnoses. Most concentrate their time on attempting to prove that a disc or bone abnormality is causing the pain. In other words, they spend all their time and energy trying to identify what comprises the cause of about ten percent of all lower back pain. Many of the so-called experts are guilty of attempting to put a square peg in a round hole. If it doesn't fit, it simply doesn't fit, but some doctors never learn that critical lesson and it is the patient that suffers. If that appears absurd to the reader, you are simply reacting in a logical, non-biased manner because it truly is absurd. A diagnosis should never be made without properly examining the patient! Knowing the anatomical structures involved is of utmost importance because that will determine what treatment to provide.

The previously described scenario is not fictitious and has occurred over and over again and will continue to occur because of the deficits in training programs for doctors. As the old saying goes, "When you go through life with a hammer in your hand, everything begins to look like a nail." A doctor only knows what he/she knows!

All other areas of the body are subject to the similar problems as I've noted with the lower back. Unfortunately, most of the accepted "experts" are no more knowledgeable about the other areas of the body than they are of the lower back. Ligaments, tendons, and joint capsules are located in every part of the body from the head to the toes. For example, I have found that most headaches as the result of an injury are the result of an injury to the neck, not the head. The original injury typically occurred in the neck (cervical spine), and then radiated to the head. Similar to lower back pain, those injuries are very common, but commonly overlooked or misdiagnosed. Again, many doctors focus on the wrong structures and dedicate their efforts toward identifying a ruptured disc or bone abnormality. Others commonly misdiagnose and call all headaches "migraines." Similar to the lower back, most pain in the neck that radiates to the head and/or the arms is the result of microscopic tearing of fibers of various support tissues. Typically, examination of those structures is overlooked, so it is no wonder that incorrect diagnoses are made.

Most patients with neck pain and headaches tell me similar stories with a few variations. In a high percentage of patients, the neck pain and headaches started as the result of an injury. It may take a number of questions asked by the doctor, because some patients with a long history of neck pain and headaches forgot when their symptoms began. Automobile accidents are very high on the list of causing that type of injury because of the tremendous forces involved. Even minor traffic accidents can take a tremendous toll on the human body. I typically discover that the neck pain started first followed by the onset of headaches, but it may not have become apparent for several days. There may be associated symptoms, such as ringing in the ears (tinnitus), increased sweating, trouble concentrating, memory impairment, anxiety, trouble sleeping, sensitivity to light, nausea, dizziness, and/or trouble swallowing. Those symptoms are commonly written off as being bizarre, but they actually describe an over-activity of the sympathetic nervous system. Two doctors by the name of Drs. Barre and Lieou described the syndrome many years ago, and the syndrome became known by the combination of their names, *Barre-Lieou Syndrome*. It is also referred to as posterior cervical sympathetic syndrome. Neurologists frequently misdiagnose these symptoms as "migraines." For most people and some neurologists, the term "migraine" is used interchangeably with headaches. That is simply incorrect, as a migraine is a headache caused by dilation of cerebral blood vessels. Most headaches, as I indicated, are the result of trauma to the neck and the headaches are caused by pain referral patterns.

The headaches originating in the neck (cervical spine) are commonly bilateral, but can be one-sided. In most cases, the headaches are on both sides with one side being more predominant. The headaches are typically located in the temporoparietal areas (side of the head), but some patients tend to describe the pain as being in the "whole head." Others describe pain behind the eyes. The severity of headaches varies greatly. The headaches are life disrupting for many patients as they are not able to continue their normal lives. Others attempt to maintain their normal lifestyle in spite of pain. The condition typically results from an injury to tissues that stabilize the facet joints in the cervical spine. There are three points at which one vertebra (spine bone) makes contact with a neighboring vertebra. The first is the disc that separates the body of one vertebra from the next. It is essentially a cushion between two bones that maintains proper alignment. The other two contact points are the facet joints. The vertebrae make contact behind the disc, one on the right and one on the left. When viewed from above, the disc and facet orientation resemble a tripod and help form a protective ring around the spinal cord. When the facet joint capsules are torn microscopically, regardless of the cause, patients will feel pain due to reasons mentioned before.

Unfortunately, the blood supply to the attachment sites of ligaments, tendons, and joint capsules is not that good, as described previously. As a result, it is not uncommon to see patients years later with pain originating from those structures because they failed to heal. Treatment is directed at promoting the healing response of those tissues. Instead of instructing a physical therapist to evaluate and treat my patient, I give precise instructions that are designed to increase blood flow to those areas. My specialty, PM&R, invented physical therapy, and it is the only specialty in medicine that trains doctors in the use of modalities that we began teaching to physical therapists many years ago. Ice massage is a very effective method and it works very well in increasing blood flow. Ice packs don't work nearly as well and I don't instruct any of my patients to waste time with ice packs unless it's simply to reduce swelling. Ice massage works in two ways. First, the cold results in a constriction of the surface blood vessels in the skin. The blood is redirected to the deeper structures or shunted. Because of the tactile stimulation of rubbing the skin with the ice, a vasoactive reflex takes place that results in dilation of deeper arterioles. Because cellular proteins are released at the site of injury that is the site where the effects of those cellular constituents are most notable. A chemical and reflex action takes place that stimulates the dilation of the arterioles and the shunted blood makes its way to the injury site bringing in needed nutrients and oxygen that stimulate the healing response. The ice massage must be performed at least six minutes each time and can be performed four to five times per day. In a more formal setting, ultrasound can also be used to stimulate the healing response by causing an attraction of cells responsible for healing, or the so-called "chemotactic reflex." That is the first line of treatment I provide for injuries to stabilize tissues that are weakened or torn. That alone works about seventy percent of the time, but if those modalities fail, I typically suggest RIT to facilitate the healing mechanism.

RIT can be used for virtually any weakened or partially torn ligament, tendon, or joint capsule that has not healed naturally or with assistance with modalities. A ligament, tendon, or capsule that is fully torn is typically a surgical issue and one that will not respond to RIT. There is recent evidence that RIT also increases growth of cartilage tissue. This has been repeatedly demonstrated in knee joints that have narrowed. A number of patients have consulted with me who had been told that the only alternative was a joint replacement because their joint space was so narrow. Many patients were told they had a "bone-on-bone" condition and the only alternative was surgery. A number of those same patients were treated with RIT in the joint space. After a few months, x-rays revealed an increase in the joint space, in many cases indicating the growth of new cartilage. Regardless of what they were told, there was an alternative, and those patients avoided expensive surgery and the risks associated with it. If a patient has a painful, non-surgical condition involving the structures identified in this chapter, then there is hope for healing and living a pain-free life with prolotherapy/RIT.

Notes

[1] Porritt, AE, "The Injection Treatment of Hydocele, Varicocele, Bursae and Naevi." Proc. Royal Society of Medicine, *Sect of Surg*, March 1931.

[2] Schultz, LW, "A treatment for subluxation of the temperomandibular joint," *JAMA* 1937; 256:1032-1035.

[3] Steindler, A. Luck, J.V., "Differential diagnosis of low back pain by procaine hydrochloride method" *JAMA*, 1938; 110:106-113.

10

HYPERBARIC OXYGEN

Our atmosphere is composed primarily of 78.08% nitrogen and 20.95% oxygen. The remaining gases are .93% argon, .036% carbon dioxide, .0018% neon, .0005% helium, .00017% methane, .0001% krypton; 00005% hydrogen, .00003% nitrous oxide, and .000004% ozone.[1] Out of all those, we all know that oxygen is the life sustaining gas in our atmosphere. Oxygen, or O^2, is the most important component of the energy producing cellular reactions. It is transported via our blood system and is designed to reach virtually every cell in the human body. We can live for weeks without food, only a few days without water, but without oxygen, we all die within minutes. That general overview helps everyone understand the obvious importance of oxygen in the hierarchy of things essential for life. When oxygen is breathed in, it attaches to hemoglobin molecules within the red blood cells. In turn, the hemoglobin is transported throughout the body where oxygen is released as needed. Once the chemical energy-producing mechanism takes place in the cell mitochondria, carbon dioxide is given off by the cells into the blood where it is then returned to the lungs and expired each time a person exhales.

One must first understand the level of importance of oxygen and the fact that it sits at the very top of the chart of ingredients that sustain life itself. By understanding this simple fact, one can then begin to develop a better understanding of how and why hyperbaric oxygen works. Hyperbaric oxygen simply means 100% oxygen given to patients with pressures greater than normal atmospheric pressure, which is almost fifteen pounds per square inch (14.7 psi actual) at sea level.

In 1674, a scientist by the name of John Mayou hypothesized that oxygen was the component of air that was involved in respiration. However, the discovery of oxygen actually did not take place until 1771. Karl Wilhelm Scheele was a Swedish chemist who made this discovery, but his printed results were delayed until 1777.[2] This led to much confusion, as another scientist, Joseph Priestly, published his results stating that he discovered oxygen in 1774. The circumstances surrounding the discovery of oxygen were subsequently investigated and it was determined that Scheele had discovered the element first. His discovery supported the hypothesis of Mayou from one hundred years before.

Once the role of oxygen became better known and accepted, spas, using compressed air (air under pressure), begin to spring up throughout Europe and were referred to as "air baths." In 1834, compressed air (hyperbaric) began being used to treat pulmonary disease. The first hyperbaric operating room was constructed in 1879, and hyperbaric air was first used to treat "nervous disorders" in the United States in 1891. It wasn't until 1937 that hyperbaric oxygen (HBO) at 100% concentration was first used in medicine. The first use was to treat decompression sickness that is more commonly known today as "the bends." A year later (1938), Brazilian doctors began treating Leprosy with hyperbaric oxygen, and American physicians began studying how HBO affected experimentally induced carbon monoxide (CO) poisoning in animals. From those experiments, it was determined that HBO treatment was life saving for patients with CO poisoning.

A very interesting and important study took place in 1959 under the guidance of Dutch cardiologist Dr. Ita Boerema. He sought to prove that hyper-oxygenated blood could result in oxygen saturation in the tissues. Indeed, he used pigs to prove his theory by removing their blood after undergoing HBO treatment at three times normal atmospheric pressure (three atmospheres). All animals will die without blood, for it is the blood that carries life sustaining oxygen to the body tissues.

His study proved that tissues saturated in oxygen, as a result of HBO treatment, remained viable for much longer than ordinary. The pigs suffered no ill effects in spite of having all their blood removed for several minutes, after which time the blood was replaced. The study was important in opening a window of opportunity for heart surgeons to operate with the heart stopped. It is as important today as it was over fifty years ago, but the heart-lung machine replaced the need for HBO before and during surgery. Dr. Boerema also discovered that HBO treatment was very effective for patients suffering from gas gangrene.

During the 1960s, it was discovered that HBO was effective in treating patients with brain ischemia (lack of blood supply), strokes, arterial occlusion in the limbs, myocardial infarctions (heart attacks), multiple sclerosis, and osteo-myelitis.[3] That list has continued to grow to the present day. In the 1960s and 1970s, the majority of HBO treatment chambers were owned and operated by the military. Gradually, the non-military medical community began to use HBO to treat various recognized conditions. It wasn't until the 1980s that structure began to develop for the certification and teaching of hyperbaric medicine. There are now a number of hyperbaric medicine organizations that are member based, and all offer guidance, education, and certification for doctors and technicians alike.

Today, there are HBO centers that are hospital based, and others are based in outlying centers that may or may not be affiliated with a hospital. Typically, the centers that are hospital based only offer treatment for conditions that are considered "labeled" traditional conditions. Labeled conditions are those that are approved by the FDA. There are many other conditions that have been shown and proven to respond very positively to HBO as well, but are still considered "off-label" because they have not been approved by the FDA. For reasons not known to me, the FDA seems to have fallen far behind in that regard. In some cases, the research studies are more convincing for many of the off-label conditions than for the labeled conditions, but it is not the intent of this book to pontificate about why beneficial treatment has not been approved by the FDA. Perhaps some of the readers of this book can make a determination in that regard. Could it be some of the same reasons that other life-saving or life-changing treatments are not recognized? The basic difference between the two categories is that labeled conditions are typically covered by health insurance because of being approved by the FDA, whereas the off-labeled conditions are not. Unfortunately, some things take an unreasonable amount of time to become accepted as being treatable by HBO. As a result, the vast majority of conditions that have proven to benefit from HBO have not been accepted and approved, so they remain off-label.

There are presently fourteen FDA approved "labeled" conditions that are typically reimbursed by insurance. They are comprised of the following:

- ❖ Decompression sickness (bends)
- ❖ Carbon monoxide poisoning and smoke inhalation
- ❖ Cyanide poisoning
- ❖ Gas gangrene
- ❖ Air or gas embolism
- ❖ Diabetic wounds
- ❖ Compromised skin grafts or flaps
- ❖ Severe anemia
- ❖ Osteomyelitis (refractory to treatment)
- ❖ Osteoradionecrosis (tissue damage secondary to radiation)
- ❖ Thermal burns
- ❖ Actinomycosis
- ❖ Crush injuries, compartment syndromes, or other traumatic ischemias
- ❖ Necrotizing soft tissue infections

The cost to treat labeled conditions with HBO varies widely and in many cases depends upon the center's contract with insurance companies. The average cost per treatment is about $800.00. If the time in the chamber is greater or the condition requires more pressure, the cost can increase.

HBO has also been proven to successfully treat "off-label" conditions as well. Off-label conditions include such maladies as:

- ❖ Strokes
- ❖ Traumatic brain injuries
- ❖ Near drowning
- ❖ Cerebral palsy
- ❖ Autism
- ❖ Brain concussions
- ❖ Seizures
- ❖ Spinal cord injuries
- ❖ Dementia
- ❖ Reflex sympathetic dystrophy
- ❖ Neuropathies
- ❖ Migraines
- ❖ ALS
- ❖ Depression
- ❖ Lyme disease
- ❖ Multiple sclerosis
- ❖ Fibromyalgia
- ❖ Interstitial cystitis
- ❖ Post-plastic surgical healing
- ❖ General wound healing or post-surgical healing
- ❖ Post-injury healing
- ❖ Macular degeneration
- ❖ Ulcerative colitis
- ❖ Crohn's disease
- ❖ Chronic fatigue syndrome
- ❖ Various infections
- ❖ Overall health

HBO treatment for off-label conditions is not covered by most insurance plans simply because the FDA has delayed matters and remains behind the times as has most of the HBO industry in regard to treating off-label conditions. The results for many of the off-label conditions are truly remarkable in many cases, but it is the patient that must pay for the treatment. Most centers offer one-hour HBO treatment sessions at a price range from $150 to $225 per treatment.

Regardless of the center being used or whether or not the condition is considered labeled or off-labeled, the treatment time is the actual time spent at the prescribed target pressure. Time is required for a patient to reach the target pressure, and additional time is required to return the patient to normal atmospheric pressure. As a result, the total time in the chamber is always greater than the time at a specific target pressure. For example, if the prescribed treatment time is one hour at depth, that means that the patient would be in the hyperbaric chamber for seventy-five to eighty minutes because of the time required to reach the prescribed pressure and the time required to return to normal atmospheric pressure. So there are no questions, treatment time is determined by the actual time at the prescribed target pressure and there are no exceptions!

Since HBO was primarily used by the military in the early days to treat decompression sickness (bends), diving terms were used and continue to be used today in HBO centers. For example, placing a patient under pressure in an HBO chamber is referred to as "diving" the patient since the pressure is the same for a person diving to certain depths in sea water. When a patient is being treated at 2.0 atmospheres, the same pressure is achieved as a diver will experience under thirty-three feet of sea water. The deeper a diver goes, the greater the pressure because of the laws of physics.

Different diseases and conditions are treated with different pressures. Brain injury conditions that respond to treatment are "off-label," as noted in many of the examples before.

Conditions such as stroke, traumatic brain injuries, and concussions are treated at 1.5 atmospheres of pressure. The optimum treatment pressures for specific conditions were determined only after treating thousands of patients at HBO centers worldwide. In our clinic, the standard pressure for treating brain injuries is 1.5 atmospheres, as noted above. However, some centers use somewhat higher pressures in an attempt to determine whether or not patients achieve a better response. Experience has shown the results from treating at higher pressures have not provided a better result. To the contrary, higher pressures typically result in a lesser response.

In order to gain some understanding of how HBO works, I will discuss treating a patient who has suffered a stroke. First, it is important to offer HBO treatment for a stroke patient as soon as they are stable. Even if HBO was being considered, treatment is typically delayed while traditional medicine provides the same rehabilitation measures they have been providing for many years. Those rehabilitation measures are definitely indicated as they are designed to help the patient achieve the best response possible. However, rehabilitation doctors worldwide are missing the boat on this issue because HBO gives the patient an even better opportunity to respond to the typical rehab treatment measures. Unfortunately, most doctors never recommend HBO for the stroke patient when, in fact, the outcome for them would be significantly improved if HBO was readily available as a part of the traditional medical model. As I indicated previously, the treatment of stroke patients is considered "off-label" and not paid for by most insurance plans. As a result, it is not made available at the time a stroke patient would get the most benefit. The majority of stroke patients come to our clinic months or years later, and usually upon the advice of a proactive, non-physician friend or family member. The earlier a patient is treated, the chance of success improves, but it is rare to treat a stroke patient at any point without seeing some improvement. One of our patients was seen after over twenty-five years had elapsed after having sustained a head injury, and three months after having sustained a stroke. Pre and post-treatment SPECT scans were obtained on this patient. The results of the scan revealed a ninety percent increase of blood flow to the traumatic brain injury area and thirty-five percent increase in the area affected by his stroke. His improvement was rather dramatic. It is important to understand that every patient is different and responds to HBO in a different manner. HBO is a viable treatment addition for these patients. It is impossible to predict the eventual outcome, but various degrees of improvement are the rules rather than the exceptions.

Strokes occur as the result of an impaired blood flow to a part of the brain. The impaired blood flow can result from an artery's interior becoming restricted because of plaque formation, as is seen in ASVD (atherosclerotic vascular disease). The problem can be compounded if a clot lodges in the area causing a cessation of blood flow to the area supplied by that vessel (occlusive). Strokes can also happen if an artery ruptures or leaks into the surrounding brain tissue (hemorrhagic) as the result of a weakened artery wall (aneurysm). When blood escapes from the vascular system into surrounding brain tissue, it results in inflammation, not to mention the fact that it causes a shift of structures as the result of occupying space normally occupied by brain tissue. The combination of factors results in dangerous swelling (edema). In the closed space of the skull, swelling can have dire immediate consequences. Bleeding can also be caused by trauma to the head and the result can be very similar to a stroke if the blood is not removed as soon as possible. The initial treatment measures for a hemorrhagic versus an occlusive stroke are entirely different and recognizing the difference can be life saving. Even if the initial treatment is successful, the patient will typically be left with some degree of neurological deficit and rehabilitation measures are typically implemented.

For proactive people who are not content to leave everything to chance, HBO is a proven viable addition. I never advise any patient to stop rehabilitation measures during HBO simply because the two work well in tandem. Stroke patients are treated at 1.5 ATA which is the equivalent of diving to 16.5 feet of seawater. That means the pressure in the chamber is one and one half times the pressure present at sea level (14.7 pounds per square inch). Patients breathe 100% oxygen, and in doing so, dissolve a significantly greater percentage of oxygen (ten to fifteen times greater) in the plasma. Diving to 1.5 atmospheres (ATA) is the equivalent of getting 150% oxygen, resulting in the red blood cells becoming super-saturated with oxygen. Strokes occur for the reasons noted above, and when blood flow ceases to a brain cell under normal temperature and pressure conditions, those cells die within just a few minutes. Nothing can revive the cells that die; however, it is known that the cells in the surrounding area (penumbral area) remain viable but dormant. "Penumbra" is a word derived from Latin and means "almost" (pen) "shadow" (umbra.) In the case of a stroke, the umbra refers to the cells that have died while the penumbra refers to the brain cells that have been placed in a dormant state due to low oxygen, but did not die because some oxygen was available. When oxygen reaches the penumbra that is, in turn, composed of dormant or so-called "idling" cells, they begin to function again.[4] Oxygen is the only thing that will activate those cells! One can begin to understand why the results in stroke patients are so varied. A larger penumbral area contains a larger amount of cells that are dormant. As those cells begin to "wake up," it results in the return of more function for that patient. One can attempt to predict how much function will return for each patient by using a SPECT scan or a PET scan, but the studies add significant additional cost. If the additional cost would prevent a patient from undergoing HBO, those studies would have to be deferred. If stroke was a labeled condition, then it would be reasonable to undergo either of those studies as a predictive indicator. However, those studies are not foolproof and are not always able to accurately predict an outcome.

HBO also stimulates growth (angiogenesis) of new capillaries (blood vessels) into the penumbra.[5] Once the cells begin functioning again, a viable blood supply must be maintained in order keep them functioning properly. HBO does just that, but it takes time for that to happen. Experience has taught us that forty one-hour treatments are necessary to accomplish the goal of capillary maturation. HBO reduces swelling as well and emphasizes why HBO should be used early on with stroke patients. For that reason alone, HBO should be an integral part every stroke rehabilitation program worldwide. Hospital based doctors have their hands tied in this regard because the "experts" have not approved HBO for use in stroke patients. How absurd is that? It is just as absurd as many of the other examples in this book, whereby so-called "experts" engage in obsolete dogmatic methods and denounce those who base their practice upon science and common sense. The reasons for HBO's non-acceptance for the treatment for a variety of off-label conditions is varied, but it comes down to the fact that many of the so-called "experts" are not experts at all. In some cases, their only expertise is protecting their turf while enriching themselves. HBO is the most effective method for treating patients who have suffered a stroke, but it remains unapproved! It makes most sane people wonder who is in charge of determining the labeled status for conditions that respond to HBO. For the inquisitive, first consider the organizations that only condone labeled conditions. Within that group, one will find a few who are concerned primarily with their position and pocketbook. Those types have been among us for centuries, and while science has made great strides in spite of them, human nature remains unchanged. If one pays close attention, it becomes rather obvious who those parties might be.

Stroke patients are observed during their treatment program for improvement in function. Their family members are also interviewed and questioned about less obvious changes taking place, such as a change in attitude, attention span, or a return of subject matter thought to be lost. After undergoing the forty treatment regimen, the patient is assessed again in regards to functional improvement, both physically and mentally. In many stroke patients, the changes are quite obvious. It is very rare not to achieve some degree of improvement. It has been speculated by doctors (typically neurologists) who criticize using HBO for stroke patients that those improvements would have taken place in the absence of HBO. When I hear that remark, I pose the question about why my patient, that had a traumatic brain injury over twenty-five years ago compounded by a more recent stroke showed such dramatic improvement with HBO? Of course, I have yet to get an answer to that question, as the critic would actually be faced with looking at the issue scientifically. Some of those doctors are simply ignorant about the subject and merely repeat what they have heard from equally ignorant colleagues instead of learning the science-based facts. My goal has been to teach willing doctors, but there is little anyone can do for the close-minded.

During 2010 and 2011, there has been a lot of talk in the media about brain concussions sustained at the time of a sports activity. Prevention is certainly the best policy, but what happens to the athlete who sustains a concussion? What treatment do they receive and how should this change? The typical "treatment" is no treatment, just observation and avoidance of any activities in which the patient could receive additional trauma to the head. The only exception to this is if the patient athlete has evidence of bleeding around the brain (subdural hematoma). That is a serious condition and should be dealt with surgically, particularly if symptoms deteriorate. However, most cases are in the "wait and see" category. Otherwise knowledgeable and educated people wait on the body's natural healing process to take place. That would be entirely acceptable if HBO was not available. However, we now know that HBO is very useful in treating post-concussion syndrome as the result of reducing swelling, promoting healing, improving the function of affected cells, and stimulating the growth of new blood vessels necessary for continued function.[6] The waiting time for returning to the sport could be reduced due to the fact that the athlete would be healthier sooner with HBO than without. Undergoing HBO certainly does not prevent further injury, but it definitely reduces the morbidity associated with that particular concussion. So why is it not used or required? Again, the dogma of medicine routinely overshadows the science of medicine. Perhaps athletes should be more proactive in this regard and demand treatment that has been proven to work, regardless of the opinions given by those who directly care for the athlete. It's the athlete's brain and the athlete's body! Keeping them both sound is in the best interest of the athlete and, indirectly, in the best interest of their whole team.

Cerebral palsy (CP) is another of the off-label conditions for which critics claim HBO is of no benefit. A similar phenomenon takes place in CP patients that occurs in stroke patients. CP results from brain cells being deprived of oxygen during or after the birth process, regardless of the reason. As with a stroke, the cells deprived of oxygen for an extended time will die and a penumbral area will develop. When the dormant cells in the penumbral area are activated with oxygen under pressure, they begin to resume activity. The resumed cellular activity can potentially cause the return of function for that patient. As with a stroke patient, the results are varied and it is impossible to predict what positive changes will take place. Those patients are also treated for forty one-hour sessions for the same reasons previously given. Patients are then advised to take a two to three month break in order to determine whether or not additional positive changes take place while their symptoms tend to stabilize. A number of patients have undergone additional forty segment treatment regimens that have helped achieve additional results. About seven or eight years ago, I witnessed one of the most remarkable outcomes achieved by a patient with cerebral palsy. The patient was an eight-year-old boy with CP who would not follow anyone or any object with his eyes (visual tracking), nor had he ever spoken a word. During the midpoint evaluation, while removing him from the chamber, he looked at his mother and said, "Love you." You could have heard a pin drop in the room and we all stood in shock until the mother's eyes filled with tears of joy. That demonstrated to me personally the potential life-changing effects of HBO for treating CP and removed any lingering doubt from my mind.

Autism is another off-label condition that has been shown to respond favorably to HBO treatment as well. The mechanism by which HBO exerts its effect does not seem to be the same as with stroke or cerebral palsy patients, but may be somewhat similar from the standpoint that the brain is thought to not get a proper supply of oxygen-rich blood.[7] It is currently believed that increased oxygen from HBO results in activation of sluggish mitochondria and reduces inflammation that results in the improvement in motivation, speech, and/or awareness.

Reflex sympathetic dystrophy also responds quite well to HBO. Every patient treated through our clinic has achieved results as evidenced by decreased swelling, decreased pain, and improved mobility. It is interesting to note that the majority of those patients were also hypothyroid.

There are a number of diseases that are referred to as collagen vascular diseases such as rheumatoid arthritis, Crohn's disease, ulcerative colitis, lupus, polymyositis, etc. They are considered auto-immune type diseases in which the body forms antibodies against its own tissues. It is suspected that these diseases are the result of an infectious agent that prospers in people with inherently weak immune systems. According to a number of sources, the infectious agent's cell wall is very similar to the tissues in the human body that are attacked by their own antibodies. As a result of the similarity, the antibodies attack the patient's tissue while the offending infectious agent hides from view by being incorporated into the host cells. It is interesting to note that many of these patients also have hypothyroidism. Unfortunately, most doctors miss the diagnosis and don't treat the underlying hypothyroidism, or under-treat it with ineffective replacement. Either way, the patients are a setup for these conditions because hypothyroidism typically results in the impairment of immune function. With reduced immune function, infectious agents are more prone to cause problems, some with disastrous consequences. With the recognition and proper treatment of hypothyroidism, it is speculated that many of these diseases would become far less common. In the interim, HBO can be used to treat each of these conditions.[8] In the case of ulcerative colitis, it has been reported that the disease is 100% responsive to HBO in achieving remission, and it is quite rare to find any treatment that is 100% effective. Regardless, why take dangerous drugs or undergo surgery when HBO can offer success in treating many of the above noted conditions?

Lyme disease is an infectious disease that is difficult to diagnose and certainly difficult to treat. The missing link for treating this serious disease has been HBO.[9] The offending infectious organism is called Borrelia burdorferi that is carried by the deer tick. The name, Lyme, originated from the town, Lyme, Connecticut, where the disease was first identified. The recommended treatment is antibiotics, but the organism can become immune to antibiotics if and when it encapsulates itself in a protein sheath or spore. When that happens, HBO serves to help dissolve the spore coat, thereby making the infectious agent susceptible to antibiotics. The typical HBO treatment program uses a pressure of 2.36 atmospheres (forty-five feet of seawater) for up to ninety minutes. It is also known that many Lyme patients have co-existing infections and those organisms must be eradicated as well. When the offending organisms are properly treated with antibiotics while the patient is undergoing HBO, the cell contents (endotoxins) are released into the patient's system, causing a symptom complex referred to as a Herx (Herxheimer) reaction. The contents of the cells are toxic and can't be removed from the system fast enough, so the patient can experience fever, chills, muscle pain, headaches, and other symptoms commonly seen with a number of other infectious diseases. After a few days, the symptoms improve as the endotoxins are removed from the patient's system. Once the infectious agent is eradicated, the remaining symptoms of Lyme disease can also be treated with HBO. It is not unusual for Lyme patients to develop neurological symptoms that can vary from mild to severe. The disease itself must be treated first, but the neurological symptoms should also be treated later in the course after the disease itself has been controlled. As with other brain conditions, HBO at 1.5 atmospheres is standard treatment for the neurological symptoms of Lyme disease and commonly results in symptom improvement as the cells begin to function normally again.

At the other end of the spectrum are non-healing sports injuries or post-surgical conditions. Those and a number of other conditions are treated at a much higher pressure of 2.36 atmospheres. As an example, studies have already been completed and published that have proven HBO to be effective for athletes with injuries. The healing time for those types of conditions is accelerated by up to seventy percent using HBO![10] It makes one wonder why every athletic facility does not have HBO available. When I hear of a famous athlete undergoing "successful" surgery for repair of an injury, I question who determined that the surgery was successful. Do you ever hear of an athlete undergoing "unsuccessful" surgery? I find it interesting that it is the surgeon that performed the surgery who states that the surgery was successful! Why have many surgeons not caught on to the fact that their surgeries would have a much higher degree of success if they would only use HBO to accelerate healing?[11] The surgeries are performed and the injuries continue to occur, but the doctors leave the healing process to mere chance! Multi-million dollar athletes sit on benches every year simply because the medical and sports community has remained in the dark ages in regards to healing. As with many other areas of medicine, the acceptance of HBO has lagged behind resulting in needless suffering, not to mention the tremendous negative financial impact.

Another issue that has resulted in confusion regarding athletic injuries being treatable by HBO has been the development of the so-called "canvas bag" chambers that are often confused with real hyperbaric oxygen chambers. A rather misleading study was published in September 1997 in the *American Journal of Sports Medicine* that concluded there was no difference in the results of treating ankle sprains with compressed air versus hyperbaric oxygen. Regardless of the reported results, the laws of physics and physiology still apply! The degree to which oxygen is dissolved in plasma (ten to fifteen times greater than normal), not to mention the oxygen tension at the cell wall, are so drastically different that one wonders about the validity of the results reported in that study. The treatment sessions were very limited (3) and actually provided little chance for noticeable changes to take place even with the significant difference in physics and physiology.[12] Why wasn't the study continued for additional treatment sessions, at which point changes would have become much more apparent? It makes one wonder about who funded the study. Was someone or some company attempting to infer that canvas bag chambers, using room air, were just as effective as HBO? That is simply not the case! Regardless of the confusion and misdirection, it would seem that the principals (managers, coaches, owners, alumni) involved would want their star players on the field instead of sitting on the bench waiting for the slower, natural healing process to take place. The situation of ignoring the healing process occurs routinely and one can see and hear proof simply by listening to the news or reading the newspaper sports section. The next time you hear about the latest famous athlete undergoing "successful" surgery, you will know who claimed it was successful and the athlete will not be receiving HBO to accelerate healing. Why?? For the same reasons medicine remains in the dark ages in other areas!

I am often asked about reports of athletes sleeping in hyperbaric chambers or treating themselves at home. That brings up the subject of discussing the two types of chambers available that I touched upon previously. The hard shell (real hyperbaric oxygen) chambers are engineered to tolerate the pressures necessary to treat any condition effectively. They are the only types of chambers authorized to use 100% oxygen. There are a variety of manufacturers that make hard chambers that meet all standards. A hard chamber is typically made of metal in combination with a very strong transparent polymer that enables the patient to see outside the chamber. This is the type of chamber found in clinics and hospitals that treat the fourteen labeled conditions. These chambers can also be found in facilities that treat off-label conditions because the chamber can achieve the pressures necessary to treat all conditions. The other type of chamber is constructed of strong nylon (or similar synthetic fiber) canvas and are referred to as soft, mild, or bag chambers. Entering and exiting are facilitated through an opening using zippers. The maximum pressure obtainable in a soft chamber is 1.3 atmospheres, and because of safety reasons, nothing other than room air is authorized for use. They are authorized for the treatment of altitude sickness only. Soft chambers are less expensive and offer some benefit for those who don't have access to a real hyperbaric oxygen (hard shell) chamber. Since the canvas chambers are limited in the pressure they can achieve and the oxygen concentration they can legally use, the conditions they can treat effectively is likewise very limited, regardless of what a few misleading "studies" claim.

Treatment with HBO is not without risk. Some patients are claustrophobic and have a fear of tight places. Chambers vary in size from twenty-five inches in diameter (monoplace) to large (multi-place) chambers with room for eight to ten people plus an attendant. The issue of claustrophobia, although rare, typically occurs only when monoplace chambers are used. Those patients are counseled and treated with anxiety reducing medications if necessary, and it usually ceases to be a problem at that point. After treating patients with HBO for over ten years, I can recall only one patient who refused treatment because of claustrophobia.

Another risk is barotrauma, or injury to the tympanic membrane (ear drum) as the result of differing pressures outside and inside the eardrum. All patients are instructed to "clear" (another diving term) their ears during the change in pressure. An attendant is always present beside the chamber to facilitate that procedure and most problems can be avoided with a skilled staff in place. Problems can arise when a patient cannot clear properly and treatment is stopped until the issue is resolved. Myringotomies, or placement of ear tubes, can be performed to equalize the pressure, thereby avoiding eardrum pressure trauma.

HBO can result in oxygen toxicity when treatment is given at higher pressures or for extended times. There are actually two types of oxygen toxicity, pulmonary and CNS (central nervous system). We treat at a maximum of 2.36 atmospheres which is the equivalent of diving to forty-five feet of seawater. We treat injured athletes, non-healing post-surgical patients, and Lyme disease at that pressure for up to ninety minutes of "down time," or the time at the maximum prescribed pressure. For those patients treated for ninety minutes, we always perform an "air break" at the halfway point. An air break is when the patient breathes normal air for five minutes, and then resumes breathing 100% oxygen for the remainder of the treatment time. Air breaks prevent CNS oxygen toxicity. The signs and symptoms of CNS toxicity are changes in vision, changes in hearing, anxiety, ringing in the ears, disorientation, and seizures. We are very observant for any signs of CNS toxicity, plus we provide air breaks for appropriate patients. As a result, oxygen toxicity has never occurred at our clinic. Pulmonary toxicity usually begins with episodes of coughing that increases in severity and can be followed by chest pain and shortness of breath. Fortunately, that phenomenon has not occurred in our center since our longest treatment time is ninety minutes and more time is necessary for the development of pulmonary toxicity. While rare, a pneumothorax can also result from the pressures reached in a hyperbaric chamber and attendants must always be aware that it can take place, regardless of how rare it is. Proper pre-screening and the presence of a skilled and attentive staff that follow proper procedures and protocol reduce the incidence of toxicity considerably.

Oxygen under pressure is extremely flammable and safety precautions are of utmost concern and importance at our clinic. A staff of highly-trained technicians should always be in place and take all necessary safety precautions. All patients should be provided appropriate gowns or scrub outfits and never be allowed to enter a chamber with any device or implement that might spark or create static electricity. Patients should never be allowed to enter a chamber wearing normal clothing.

In summary, treatment with HBO is recognized as being effective for many conditions that, heretofore, had no options in regard to treatment. Fourteen conditions are approved by the FDA and insurance pays for those conditions. Those are considered "labeled" conditions. However, many conditions remain unapproved "off-label" in spite of proven efficacy. Those conditions are not reimbursable under most insurance plans so patients or their families must be proactive in that regard. Many off-label conditions will be granted approval once enough attention and pressure is brought to bear upon those who are in the position to make said approval take place. At this point, it is the patient who must seek and pay for HBO treatment for those conditions. Most doctors know little about HBO and its treatment for recognized conditions, so why assume they would know about the treatment of "off-label" conditions? Again, what your doctor doesn't know can hurt you!

Notes

[1] Pedwirny, M. "Atmospheric Composition," *Fundamentals of Physical Geography, Second edition*, 2006.

[2] *Journal of the American Medical Association Vol. 212, no. 13*; June 29, 1970, 2258-2259.

[3] Neubauer, R. and Walker, M.; *Hyperbaric Oxygen*, Penguin Putnam Inc., New York, 1998.

[4] Neubauer,R.A. et al, "Enhancing "idling" neurons," *Lancet*, 335:542, 1990

[5] Siddiqui, A. et al, "Ishemic tissue oxygen capacitance after hyperbaric oxygen therapy: new physiological concept," *Plastic Reconstructive Surgery*, 1997;99(1):148-155.

[6] Eltorai, I., Montroy, R., "Hyperbaric Oxygen Therapy Leading to Recovery of a 6-week Comatose Patient Afflicted by Anoxic Encephalopathy and Posttraumatic Edema," *J. Hyperbaric Med.* 1991; 6(3), 189-198.

[7] Rossignol, D., "Hyperbaric oxygen therapy might improve certain pathophysiological findings in autism," *Medical Hypothesis* (2097) 68, 1208-1227.

[8] Buckman, A.L. et al, "Hyperbaric oxygen therapy for severe ulcerative colitis," *J Clin Gastroenterol.* 2001 Oct; 33(4):337-339.

[9] Fife, W., *Effects of Hyperbaric Oxygen Therapy on Lyme Disease*, Texas A&M Univ., Jan 29, 1998.

[10] James P.B. et al, "Hyperbaric Oxygen Therapy in Sports Injuries"; *Physiotherapy, volume 9, no. 8*, August 1993.

[11] Gunalp U et al, "Hyperbaric Oxygen Therapy as an Adjunct to Surgical Treatment of Extensive Hidradenitis Suppurativa"; *World Journal of Surgery, Vol. 34, No. 4*, 861-862

[12] Borromeo C.N. et al: Hyperbaric oxygen therapy for acute ankle sprains; *American Journal of Sports Medicine*, 1997; 25(5): 619-625

11

BLINKING LIGHTS, BELLS, AND WHISTLES

Beginning with the Preface of this book, I alluded to the fact that many doctors practice medicine in a manner that often leaves common sense behind. As doctors, we are taught many things that are supposedly science-based. In fact, I have provided a number of examples wherein doctors simply repeat what they've learned and never question the authenticity of the commonly accepted standard of care. In many of the examples provided, the accepted "facts" are not always based upon science; to the contrary, myth and pseudoscience are common ingredients in twenty-first century medicine. Our contemporary medical model is based upon the treatment of disease symptoms with little interest or attempts to prevent those diseases or treat the causes. **Most doctors truly have their patients' best interests and optimal health in mind.** However, the doctors' frames of reference have been distorted by faulty or incomplete training to the extent that some of what they learned is actually detrimental to their patients' health. Many doctors are simply ignorant (uninformed) about some of the issues pointed out in this book, but a problem arises if and when a doctor refuses to learn when faced with scientific facts. Of course, there will always be the ones who will remain members of the "flat earth society," regardless of how many facts are available. As with any profession, medicine has its share of less competent members that are bound to do harm, regardless of their specialty. The overwhelming majority of doctors are competent, but can still harm patients simply because their training has been incomplete in a number of vitally important areas mentioned in this book. Each and every one of those doctors has the opportunity to learn additional readily available and known methods of optimizing their patients' health. The doctors who choose not to be confused with scientific facts by being arrogant and close-minded, regardless of the reason, should question their motives for entering the honored profession of medicine in the first place.

In spite of many technical advances, doctors remain confused and uncertain about the causes of many conditions and illnesses. Time will eventually reveal that present day doctors had only begun to scratch the surface about revelations and mind-boggling discoveries yet to come during the next hundred or so years. That progress will happen, but it will not be because of the doctors who stubbornly and dogmatically adhered to pseudoscientific rumors and myths. It will happen because a few innovative and courageous doctors and scientists will seek real answers to many aspects of medicine that are still in the dark ages. Consider the abject failure of the **"war on cancer."** The only way that "war" will be won is to investigate all promising treatment measures, even when they don't comply with the multi-decade failed method of incorporating the triad of surgery, radiation, and/or chemotherapy. Unfortunately, many science-based doctors have been harassed with fines, the loss of their licenses, or imprisonment simply because they sought more scientifically logical approaches to treating cancer. It is the twenty-first century, but we remain far behind in regard to treating this vicious malady. Why has this happened and why does there seem to be so much resistance to actually finding a cure? It's reasonable to assume that honorable and sensible people want to find a cure for all cancers. As I indicated in another chapter, if one truly wants the answer to why the treatment for cancer has not changed appreciably during the last sixty-plus years, it would be wise to consider the companies and individuals who have the most to gain by continuing this ill-fated "war." The treatment for cancer is archaic and it does not work in the vast majority of cases! Many of those resistant to change are the same individuals or companies that speak against prevention as well, but patients still have a choice of how and where to be treated. The failure of the "war on cancer" has also created an atmosphere that is favorable for unscrupulous scam artists who offer fraudulent remedies. Those that promote fraudulent methods are simply crooks and should be dealt with accordingly. The problem arises when attempting to decide what is bogus and what is not. As noted above, instead of continuing this ill-fated, unsuccessful war, efforts should be directed toward discovering authentic treatment methods for this terrible scourge. In order for this to take place, persecution and intimidation of innovative scientists must stop and be replaced by investigational support.

Consider the impact and result of what would happen if a "cure" for all cancers was actually discovered and *made available*. All fund-raising efforts would cease as there would no longer be a necessity. Many of the present day fund-raising organizations would close their doors if a cure was discovered. The necessity for using dangerously toxic chemotherapeutic agents would cease. A reasonable person would have to consider who makes those outrageously expensive chemotherapeutic agents and who profits by their continued use. Those companies would sustain a significant loss of profits. Would there be any objections raised by those companies if the cure was found? Does that mean that the employees of those companies are bad people? Of course not, but many become desensitized and close their minds to finding a real cure. The need to irradiate would also cease and radiation oncologists would have to either change careers or resume other aspects of radiology. Oncology surgeons would also be out of the cancer business, but could maintain a viable practice performing surgery for non-cancerous conditions. Another obvious group that would stand to lose would be the specialists in the field of oncology. Once the cure is discovered, if it already has not been, oncologists would most likely be the first to step forward and claim to have discovered the cure, even though they are the very group that has been adamantly opposed to alternative treatment methods for cancer. The above mentioned groups are the obvious potential losers if the cure is discovered, but what about the tremendous financial windfall that would occur for the patients and families whose lives are saved? Essentially, the cure would keep the afflicted away from death's door as the diagnosis of cancer would no longer be a death sentence. Our economy would be stimulated tremendously as the result of having a more productive and a healthier work force. Days lost would decrease dramatically and that would result in increased production, less sick days, less insurance costs, and ultimately, tremendous savings for the entire country. Market factors would force the lowering of life and health insurance rates as the most economically devastating plague of modern man, cancer would be gone. As the result of the obvious financial savings, more effort could be directed to solving other pressing problems. The problem with the "war on cancer" is that it is going nowhere! It is a multi-billion dollar industry that enriches those who continue this charade while downplaying efforts made to actually find the cure. I wish to repeat that the people involved are not evil, most are doing the very best they can with the limited tools available.

Non-adherence to scientific principles (pseudoscience) is pervasive and involves many areas of medicine. However, when faced with scientific evidence, the true scientists must shed their bias and adopt a more science-based approach, even if that approach doesn't agree with commonly accepted medical dogma. True science-based doctors owe that to themselves and their patients. It is imperative to separate fact from fiction so that medicine can progress. That points out one of the major problems when assessing diagnostic and treatment methods. As doctors, we are all exposed to the same information during our training. By this point, the reader understands that everything we are taught is not always correct. Finding correctness in the present day medical world is a daunting task even for physicians. Once a doctor begins to analyze everything scientifically and critically, the task becomes somewhat easier, but it still requires effort.

Some within the health care community prey upon unsuspecting patients and make outrageous and bogus claims about various diagnostic and treatment methods. By using scientific buzz words and other medical jargon, they appeal to those who are looking for other approaches to a multitude of problems, including the treatment of cancer. Many patients become victims of these charlatans out of desperation. While many claim a scientific basis for their method, it is wise for patients to engage in due diligence when in doubt. When you hear of a miraculous cure that has been suppressed, or was recently discovered again after centuries of falling into obscurity, it is most likely fraudulent.

Hucksters and con-artists have been blights on society for centuries. Present day medicine is no exception, but how is an unsuspecting patient supposed to know? The distinction between fact and fiction becomes somewhat obscure. The internet is full of false claims about a variety of diagnostic and treatment methods. As an example, I have heard many stories about conditions or diseases being diagnosed using **"applied kinesiology."** Don't confuse the term with kinesiology because kinesiology is a true science that studies bodily movement facilitated by muscles and joints. As I indicated earlier, the inclusion of scientific terms is the key to many bogus claims. I personally witnessed a demonstration of this questionable method many years ago and remain of the opinion that "applied kinesiology" is purely pseudoscience and belongs in the realm of palm reading. A patient could be exposed to an equal amount of science (none) offered by coin operated fortune telling machines! There is no scientific explanation for how this smoke and mirrors operation works because the molecules of the various substances being tested do not magically or in any other way inhibit the strength or disrupt the balance of the person being tested. The proponents of this scam engage in "testing" that will show an impairment of strength or a loss of balance simply by the way the maneuver is performed. This example is only one of the bogus pseudoscience methods being taught to unsuspecting doctors. In my opinion, it is simply nonsense!

In 1852, Dr. William Carpenter described a phenomenon that he called "ideomotor action."[1] In simple terms, it meant that people tend to provide muscle movements in response to suggestion or a preconceived notion. In most cases, movements occur unconsciously. When that happens as predicted, it lends credibility to such things as applied kinesiology and puts innocent and unsuspecting people in the position of proving pseudoscientific methods. Many times, it is a case of educated people falling for a scam resulting from suggestion or an anticipated outcome. As a result, acceptance of this type of nonsense gives alternative medicine a bad name and scares doctors away from using alternative methods that are science-based and hold promise. I don't intend to mention every bogus diagnostic and treatment method, as the space requirement would be massive. However, I will mention a few others simply to alert the reader that such things exist.

I have made an observation and reached the conclusion that people (including doctors) seem to believe a device is legitimate when it has blinking lights, bells, and/or whistles. The more of each, the more believable! I assume that doctors only believe in devices that have extra bells and whistles. Of course, I'm being facetious, but again, otherwise highly educated individuals are falling for pseudoscience. If it blinks, whistles, and rings, due diligence is in order. I have looked at many devices that were being sold for the purpose of reducing pain. A number of explanations were provided as to how and why the devices worked, but it was typically scientific jargon intended to cause confusion. I have experienced neck and upper extremity pain for many years resulting from an injury to my neck over thirty years ago. I can assure anyone that I would be aware if my pain resolved or was reduced as the result of using any device. In every case, I inquired about the mechanism of action, and once the mystical realm was mentioned, I knew I was dealing with a scam artist. Phrases such as "redirecting energy fields," "changing the polarity of the molecules," and other similar, equally nonsensical verbiage is typically used. Regardless, I allowed a number of devices to be used on me and I never achieved any result! There are many of those devices available and I have yet to find one that actually measured up to the claims made. I am always amused by the devices that don't touch the skin and claims are made that energy is being directed at the source of pain. It conjured up the image of the ray gun used by Flash Gordon. Other than microwave or shortwave diathermy, I am not aware of any energy source capable of being directed to the source of pain. Those are the most questionable devices that have absolutely no scientific basis, but their promoters are cashing in. Other pain reducing devices fall within the realm of transcutaneous nerve stimulators (TENS), but because of the added blinking lights, whistles, and bells, they cost many times more. TENS units have a scientific basis and do result in varying degrees of pain relief. In spite of some devices simply being an overpriced TENS unit, other false and misleading information was provided as to how they worked. As with all questionable devices, a number of scientific buzz words and/or phrases are scattered throughout the product literature or used during a sales presentation. Again, due diligence is in order when looking at any device of that sort. Don't confuse those "pain-reducing" devices with medical devices that can actually be explained using real science. Such things as therapeutic ultrasound, microwave diathermy, TENS, intermittent traction, etc. are treatment methods that do exactly what they claim because they are all based upon science. For each, the mechanism of action has been studied, discussed, and explained using terms that are not confusing and do not conjure up the world of mysticism.

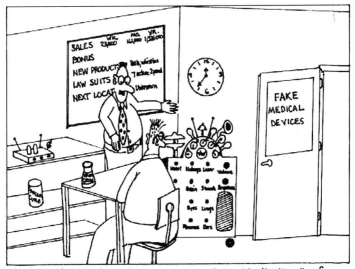

Jenkins, this is the best thing we've ever invented and by the time they figure out it does NOTHING, we'll be gone!

I attended a medical conference a number of years ago and approached a booth in which a number of people (mostly doctors) were sitting with their feet immersed in water. Of course, my curiosity got the best of me and I inquired as to what they were doing. I was told that everyone had their feet in an ionic water bath that was resulting in detoxifying though their feet. I must have looked like a deer in the headlights when I heard that, but just to investigate further, I sat down and placed my feet in one of the ionic baths. I never understood the supposed mechanism because the explanations made absolutely no sense whatsoever. The water changed from the normal appearance of water to a dark brown color. I was advised that the bath was removing a number of toxins from my body as well as parasites. To this day, I have yet to understand how those "parasites" and toxins made it all the way to my feet and then swam or oozed out in the brown water. That is one of the most absurd things I have ever heard explained, and even more unbelievable, it took place at a well-known medical conference! In reality, the water changes color as a result of the oxidation of metal electrodes that the company is willing to repeatedly sell you every time the existing electrodes oxidize and cease to function. Obviously, they cease to function as noted by their inability to oxidize and turn the water brown. The only thing in the water is iron oxide (rust), not toxins, parasites, etc.[2] In spite of the absence of scientific evidence supporting the claims for these bogus devices, they continue to be sold!

As alluded to in the chapter on human growth hormone (hGH), scam artists outnumber the legitimate internet sites. Creams, gels, and sprays, supposedly containing hGH, simply do not work for raising a patient's level of hGH, regardless of the scientific buzz words used! I reviewed a number of these products over the years and how they supposedly worked. I found them all to be bogus! The reason is that the hGH molecule is too large to be absorbed through the skin or mucous membranes. On another note, I was approached by a sales person several years ago who advised me that his company had discovered the secret to being able to apply a cream-based secretagogue to the skin that caused hGH levels to increase. To reiterate, a secretagogue for hGH simulates the pituitary to release more hGH than normal. He promised to send me the scientific evidence from trials that had established the mechanism of action and conclusively showed positive results. If it had worked, I would have definitely been interested, but it eventually became quite clear that no legitimate studies had ever been performed as claimed by the salesman. That was over fifteen years ago and I'm still waiting on the corroborative studies! Believe it or not, that scenario is not uncommon because the cost of authentic hGH has escalated to the point that many people simply can't afford it, which leads them to find other ways to obtain the same results. Scam artists never fail to step up to fill the void!

Chelation therapy is an area of interest that deserves further investigation. I am acquainted with a number of doctors who perform chelation therapy in their respective offices for the treatment of atherosclerotic vascular disease (ASVD). In most cases, doctors claim that chelation therapy works as noted by improvement of symptoms such as chest pain, shortness of breath, and exercise tolerance. Chelation with EDTA (ethylene diamine tetraacetic acid) is FDA approved for the removal of toxic heavy metals, but it is the use of chelation for ASVD that has been questioned and remains controversial. A study has been undertaken by the National Center for Complementary and Alternative Medicine (NCCAM) that is due to be completed by 2012.[3] Provided the study is of proper design and control, it should finally resolve the issue as to whether or not chelation therapy is effective for treating coronary artery disease in particular and peripheral vascular disease generally.

Most either know or have heard of someone using magnet therapy for pain relief. Claims have been made that magnetic therapy benefits other conditions such as arthritis, diabetes, high blood pressure, cancer, fatigue, diarrhea, bed sores, and immune function as the result of "increasing blood flow" by correcting a "magnetic deficiency." Magnetic deficiency? During all my years of training and practice, I never knew that anyone could have a magnetic deficiency. The reason I never learned that is because it's a false claim. Furthermore, there is no increased blood flow that results from the use of static magnets placed on the skin. In my opinion, it's another case of using scientific sounding jargon to promote a questionable treatment method at the consumer's expense. Perhaps a legitimate properly designed study will take place and put an end to the controversy, but presently, there is no legitimate **well-designed** scientific study to support the claims that magnets applied to the skin, magnetized water, mattresses, or chairs provide any documented benefit. A study completed at Baylor University and published in 1997 dealt with knee pain in patients who had been infected with the polio virus when they were children. Magnets were applied to the skin of the knees of twenty-nine patients and a sham (fake) magnet was placed on the knees of twenty-one other patients. According to the results of the study, the twenty-nine patients using the static magnet (treatment group) achieved more pain relief than the twenty-one using the non-magnetized metal piece (control group).[4] The study was flawed because the two groups were not equal in a number of ways. First, the ratio of women to men in the treatment group was twice that of the control group. If the ratio of women to men had been equal, the result would have been much more credible. It has been speculated that women are more prone to the placebo effect (suggestion) than men. Therefore, the treatment group that contained a significantly higher percentage of women would be expected to report a positive result. The power of suggestion is very powerful and the placebo (inert substance) response is alive and well in the field of magnet therapy. In order to assess a pain response, patients were asked to rate the pain elicited when a "trigger point" was touched. Was the pressure for all trigger point testing the same for every patient? If so, how was that measured? In summary, the study could have been designed in a manner that would have allowed a comparison of similar patient populations and the variable for the pressure used when testing trigger points could have been standardized as well. Perhaps the study should be repeated with those variables removed. Another study was published in 2003 about patients with painful diabetic neuropathies treated with magnetic insoles or nonmagnetic insoles. Each of the 259 patients was randomly assigned to either a treatment or control group. The authors concluded that there was a statistically significant reduction of tingling, numbness, burning, and exercise-induced pain in the treatment group as compared to the control group. They indicated there was only a modest clinical benefit. In order to further analyze whether or not the conclusions from both studies were valid, it is important to consider the results of studies that concluded that there is no evidence to support the claim that static magnets are effective in relieving or reducing pain. Accordingly, a review of twenty-nine relevant studies about static magnets was undertaken and the results were published in 2007. After scientific review of the twenty-nine studies, it was concluded, "The evidence does not support the use of static magnets for pain relief, and therefore magnets cannot be recommended as an effective treatment."[5] In summary, it appears that there is no authentic evidence to recommend magnetic therapy for pain relief or any of the other maladies mentioned.

Is there any scientific basis to support the use of copper bracelets as an effective treatment for arthritis? There are many stories claiming miraculous results from wearing a copper bracelet, but they do not stand up to scientific scrutiny. It is well known that the skin can absorb heavy metals such as lead and mercury. Copper can also be absorbed, but the amount absorbed is so miniscule that it would make little or no difference. When ingested, copper has an antioxidant effect, so there may be some credibility to the reports of people achieving some reduction of arthritis pain when wearing a bracelet, but it is not a cure, nor will one obtain a complete reduction of pain unless that pain was very minor. Since a pure copper bracelet is non-toxic and won't cause any ill effect, there is no harm in wearing a bracelet, particularly if the individual likes copper jewelry. The only exception is if the person is allergic to copper or if there are other contaminants in the composition of the bracelet such as lead.

Coral calcium was a buzz word for a number of years and unrealistic claims were made regarding its effects. False claims were made that it was effective for treating cancer and a number of other conditions. As a result, substantial fines were levied and the manufacturers were placed on notice to refrain from making any further false claims. Coral calcium is primarily calcium carbonate and is no different than calcium carbonate from other sources. There is no problem consuming appropriate doses of calcium carbonate derived from coral (other than the expense), particularly when an individual is deficient in calcium. A potential problem arises if pollutants are a part of coral calcium and are not removed. Otherwise, health problems could develop and would be no different than ingesting pollutants from any source. For example, coral off the coast of Okinawa is known to have high levels of mercury and lead, which has resulted in the concern that a higher probability of contaminated coral calcium may exist. Calcium carbonate from sources other than coral is less expensive and equally effective. It can be purchased at most stores that offer nutritional supplements.

Seasilver is a liquid multimineral, multivitamin, and amino acid product that was initially marketed through doctors' offices beginning in the 1980s. In 1994, the distribution system was restructured and the product was subsequently sold through independent multi-level marketing distributors. Unsubstantiated and outrageous claims were made about the product's effectiveness in treating a variety of diseases and conditions including cancer. Other claims were made that Seasilver purified the blood and immune systems, oxygenated body cells, strengthened the immune system, balanced body chemistry, and protected tissues and cells against "challenges." The foregoing is a prime example of using medical terminology to exploit and confuse the uninformed and naïve. That is the hallmark of pseudoscience promoting a product with little actual value. In June 2003, the FTC charged the company with deceptive marketing as the result of making unsubstantiated safety and disease claims. The Nevada Federal Court found in favor of the FTC and issued an immediate restraining order against the defendants that prohibited marketing or selling their product without substantial changes to their labeling and marketing materials. The court also issued an order prohibiting all claims of benefit unless those claims were substantiated by competent and reliable scientific evidence. The court also froze all company assets derived from the sale of the Seasilver product and over $7.8 million dollars worth of product was seized and destroyed. The company was permitted to resume marketing their product in

October 2003 after it was determined that all stipulations, issued by the court, had been met. A fine of $120 million dollars was also levied against the company and its principals, but that was subsequently reduced.[6] In spite of the punitive actions brought about as the result of deceptive marketing and false claims, the company is still selling its concoction.

Opportunists and con artists are very good at bilking the public and doctors out of millions of dollars by selling them a variety of products that have little or no legitimate function. The only scenario that would be any worse would be selling the same products while killing unsuspecting people as well. Believe it or not, that happens routinely, but instead of referring to them as quacks, they are known as pharmaceutical companies. If a nutraceutical (nutritional supplement) company marketed a vitamin or mineral that resulted in the death of just one person, the outcry would be deafening. Why do the same groups not label the pharmaceutical company principals as being quacks or perpetrators of fraud? Is that a double standard? Why not assign the same label to all offenders?

Before I give examples of egregious behavior engaged in by some in the pharmaceutical industry, I wish to make something very clear. **I do not have a vendetta against pharmaceutical companies; to the contrary, they have been responsible for developing many new drugs that have benefitted millions of people.** In order to bring pharmaceuticals to the market place, they have to spend literally millions of dollars in research, development, marketing, packaging, and distribution. I have absolutely no problem with the pharmaceutical industry bringing new drugs to the marketplace, provided they do not harm the people taking those drugs. However, they cross the line if and when they distort the truth and attempt to cover-up or not disclose information concerning the disastrous and sometimes fatal consequence of taking a particular product.

A number of pharmaceutical companies have reaped millions in profits while killing or maiming people. I have a number of examples, but I will first mention the drug, Vioxx®. It is one of the so-called non-steroidal anti-inflammatory drugs (NSAIDs) and known more specifically as a COX II inhibitor. It was approved for sale in 1999. From 1999 through September 2004, the FDA estimated that Vioxx resulted in the deaths of almost 28,000 patients. I repeat, the FDA *reported* that almost **28,000** patients died as the result of taking Vioxx. My opinion is that it is conceivable that the death toll was much higher than the estimate proposed by the very agency that is supposed to protect the American public. It was pulled from the market in September 2004 because of pressure from outside sources. Unbelievably, the manufacturing company had knowledge of serious problems with Vioxx as early as 2000, but they continued to sell it until 2004. Not only did they not remove the drug from the market, but they attempted to cover up the results by distorting the results of studies.[7] Dr. Richard Horton, editor of a prestigious medical journal (*The Lancet*) stated, "The licensing of Vioxx and its continued use in the face of unambiguous evidence of harm have been public health catastrophes. This controversy will not end with the drug's withdrawal. Merck's likely litigation bill was estimated to be as much as $50 billion.[8] The obvious question is; **why did the FDA approve Vioxx in the first place?** The drug was approved **because the FDA does not do the job it is supposed to be doing.** It's ironic that the FDA gears up if a nutritional supplement is thought to be tainted, but fail to withhold drugs like Vioxx that have serious and even fatal consequences.

In spite of the many lives lost as the result of the preventable Vioxx tragedy, the same thing could happen again because the FDA really does not appear to protect the public. On August 30, 2005, an interview was conducted with Dr. David Graham, a senior drug safety researcher for the FDA. The interview was conducted by Manette Louden. In that interview, Dr. Graham was asked about previous comments made by him regarding whether or not the FDA was capable of protecting the public against another Vioxx. His reply was,

"Since November, when I appeared before the Senate Finance Committee and announced to the world that **the FDA was incapable of protecting from unsafe drugs or from another Vioxx, very little has changed** on the surface and substantially **nothing has changed.** The structural problems that exist within the FDA, where the people who approve the drugs are also the ones that oversee the post marketing regulation of the drug, remain unchanged. The people who approve a drug when they see that there is a safety problem with it are very reluctant to do anything about it because it will reflect badly upon them. **They continue to let the damage occur. America is just as at risk now, as it was in November, as it was two years ago, and as it was five years ago."** Dr. Graham went on to say, "When there are unsafe drugs, the FDA is likely to err on the side of industry...**Safety flaws are discovered after the drug gets on the market."**[9]

The message, gleaned from Dr. Graham's interview, was that the FDA seems to be more concerned with whether or not a drug fulfills its purpose and less with safety issues. That is mind boggling considering the fact that a government agency (FDA) is charged with protecting the public. It is quite obvious that it is far more important to protect life than it is to ensure the potency or effect of a drug. There is something very wrong with that picture, but the bureaucrats at the FDA, in my opinion, seem to be more interested in protecting their own turf as opposed to the very lives of the citizens they are supposed to protect. It certainly does little to instill confidence and forces us all to wonder when the next killer drug will be approved and used on the unsuspecting public. Australian courts ruled that Vioxx should have never been approved and allowed on the market.[10]

Another drug similar to Vioxx was Bextra. It was another COX II inhibitor and caused similar problems noted with

Vioxx, with an increased incidence of heart attack and stroke as well as the development of fatal skin condition known as Stevens Johnson Syndrome. Since it was on the market for a shorter period of time, the number of deaths attributable to Bextra was far less than that caused by Vioxx. The drug remained on the market for only one year and was withdrawn in 2005. The obvious question again is, why did the FDA allow the drug to be approved when the risks were well known? The manufacturer and distributor of the drug paid out almost $2 billion to settle cases brought against them because of Bextra.

The hugely popular weight loss drug Fen-Phen (fenfluramine/phentermine) was on the market and pre-scribed to the unsuspecting public for twenty-four years before being recalled in 1994. Its popularity peaked during the 1990s. When it became evident that people were suffering serious heart and lung problems, leading to death in many cases, as a result of taking Fen-Phen for weight loss, the FDA recalled the drug. It has been estimated that over 50,000 patients filed suit against the manufacturer that cost them up to $21 billion when combined with their own legal expenses.

Baycol (cerivastatin) was a cholesterol lowering drug. A number of cholesterol lowering agents have been manufactured and made available as a result of the pseudoscience surrounding the myth that cholesterol causes heart disease. In the case of Baycol, it was discovered that it caused a severe muscle disorder called rhabdomyolysis that results in the destruction of muscle tissue. As a result of deteriorating muscle tissue, excessive protein caused irreparable kidney damage leading to over **100,000 deaths.** Yes, you read that right, **100,000 deaths!** It was recalled in 2001 after being on the market four years. The company ended up paying damages of $1.2 billion. Why did the FDA allow this drug to make it to the market? My advice is to think twice before taking any cholesterol-lowering agent, regardless of how many times it makes an appearance on a television commercial. Nice marketing, but not great drugs, especially given the fact that it has NEVER been proven that high cholesterol causes heart disease.

The foregoing are only a few examples of drugs that have been removed from the market, but there will be more. What is it going to take for the FDA to actually perform their job properly and protect the American public? Public outcry? Probably not! Congressional hearings? Maybe!

The last examples were given in order to draw attention to the fact that fraud also takes place within successful and respected companies. While two wrongs don't make a right, as the old saying goes, one needs to understand that it is not just the common con man who perpetrates fraud. Fraud is fraud, but there are degrees. When anyone engages in fraud with the intent of personal enrichment by taking money for devices or methods that have no scientific basis, that definitely demonstrates a lack of character and conscience on the part of the con man. Those types will always be within our midst and should be avoided, exposed, and prosecuted. Some of the initial examples were of that variety. In those cases, most people don't die or get sick; they are simply cheated out of their money. The exception to that are the perpetrators of fraud who promote ineffective cancer cures. The cases of dangerous drugs being brought to market are the most egregious of the lot. That is fraud, but it is accompanied by death and maiming. There seems to be a double standard in regards to the perpetrators of fraud. Fraud is no less when it is perpetrated by a large company. It would seem logical to place those companies at the top of the quack list issued by groups who claim to have the goal of protecting the unsuspecting public from fraud. The next time you check out one of those groups, I think one might be very surprised to find the absence of those names who are perpetrating the most unbelievable fraud that should rank at the top of the list. If those self-appointed groups are going to protect us all from fraud in a forthright manner for altruistic reasons, then by all means do it by naming the very worst offenders before worrying so much about others that pale in comparison.

Notes

[1] Carpenter, WB, "On the influence of suggestion in modifying and directing muscular movement independent of volition." *Proceedings of the Royal Institution of Great Britain*, 1852:147-153.

[2] Weil, A, DrWeil.com, Questions and Answers; Feb. 20, 2007

[3] NCCAM.nih.gov; Questions and Answers:The NIH Trial of EDTA Chelation Therapy for Coronary Artery Disease.

[4] Vallbona c. et al, "Response of pain to static magnetic fields in post polio patients: A double-blind pilot study." *Archives of Physical and Rehabilitative Medicine*, 1997, 78:1200-1203.

[5] Pittler MH et al, "Static magnets for reducing pain: systematic review and meta-analysis of randomized trials." *Canadian Medical Association Journal*, Sept 2007, 177(7):736-742.

[6] "Marketers of Seasilver agree to pay 4.5 million to settle FTC charges." FTC news release, March 17, 2004.

[7] Adams, M., "Merck caught in scandal to hide Vioxx heart attack risks, intimidate scientists and keep pushing dangerous drugs; Vioxx lawsuits now forming." NaturalNews.com. November 6, 2004.

[8] The Manhattan Law Institute's Trial Lawyers, Inc.:Healthcare report. 2005.

[9] Loudon, M., "The FDA Exposed: An Interview with Dr. David Graham, the Vioxx Whistleblower." August 30, 2005.

[10] Huff, Ethan A., "Australian courts rule that Vioxx should have never been approved for sale." NaturalNews.com., June 20, 2010.

12

HEALTH HAZARDS EXPOSED

Chemistry has assisted mankind in many ways, but it has also helped create compounds that are unhealthy, dangerous, and sometimes deadly. We are exposed to chemical pollutants and toxins in our air, soil, food, water, homes, clothing, automobiles, cosmetics, cleaning products, and the list goes on and on. We are, for the most part, unable to avoid pollutants and toxins regardless of where we live and work. That's truly a scary thought, but it is possible to reduce some of those threats simply by becoming aware. It has been estimated that over 72,000 new chemicals have been developed since World War II, and have made their way to the marketplace. That equates to just under 1,100 new chemicals entering our environment every year for the last sixty-six years! Many of those are toxic to humans and it is wise to know the ones we can avoid, eliminate, or reduce. The unfortunate part of this scenario is that less than two percent of these chemicals have been tested as a cause of toxicity, cancer, or birth defects in humans. In other words, out of the almost 1,100 new chemicals added to our environment each year, about 1,069 are not tested for toxicity! Incredible as that may sound, it is true. Accordingly, we must all become proactive in an attempt to protect ourselves, our families, and our friends from hazards that are known. Something is extremely wrong with our environment; otherwise, the death rate from cancer would be decreasing. Since 1960, it has been estimated that cancer rates have almost doubled. So much for the "war on cancer!" With so many known chemical carcinogens in our environment, and considering the fact that so few newly released chemicals are tested properly, it is logical to assume that many of these chemicals are contributing to or causing many of the devastating health problems that are so commonplace today. Cancer is now the number one killer of children! That is a sobering thought indeed. The most innocent members of our society are being taken from us before they have a chance to live a full and productive life!

One doesn't have to visit a chemical plant in order to be exposed to pollutants and toxic chemicals. In some cases, the toxic environment of those plants might actually be less toxic than one's home. An EPA survey concluded that the air in a home is from three to seventy times more polluted than the outside air! We lock ourselves inside our energy efficient homes with toxic chemicals being released into the environment! As a result, one must become aware of toxins in your own home that reside on your shelves, in your closets, garage, and basement. Once one becomes aware, then the avoidance or elimination process can begin. Some are very obvious and are known to be toxic, so I don't intend to spend a great deal of time and effort talking about gasoline, motor oil, solvents, paint, pesticides, and cleaning compounds. Household cleaning solutions are the number one cause of poisoning in children. OSHA found over 2,500 chemicals in cosmetics that were toxic, and most people have little if any knowledge about that issue. There are lesser known toxins in other areas of the home as well and some of those will be discussed. It has been estimated that every home contains at least sixty two toxic chemicals! Is there any wonder why asthma, cancer, skin diseases, and behavioral problems in children have skyrocketed?

When I was in elementary school in the 1950s, it was rare that children were medicated for attention deficit hyperactivity disorders (ADHD). As a matter of fact, I can't recall even **one** instance of that happening, unless it was a well kept secret! Have you ever known kids to keep secrets? It is now routine for children to be medicated. Is it because we are now able to make the diagnosis, whereas before we didn't have the intelligence to determine that a child had a behavioral problem? I remember most children sitting in their seats until given permission to leave class. Other than some minor disruption, that was typical. So ask yourself, why has this major behavioral change taken place? I believe, as do many experts, that the escalation of behavioral problems, the increased incidence of asthma **(600% increase since 1980),** and the increased rate of cancers are due to the toxicity we are exposed to everyday. Since many chapters in this book deal with hormonal issues, I would be remiss not to mention that environmental pollutants and toxins can exert a tremendous impact upon our endocrine system. Since most chemicals are not properly studied, it is virtually impossible to keep up with how every chemical affects our endocrine system and hormones. If one has a known hypersensitivity to any chemical, it is logical to remove that chemical from your home or work place. The Environmental Protection Agency (EPA) has estimated that thirty percent of insecticides, sixty percent of herbicides, and ninety of fungicides are known to be carcinogenic. The problem is knowing which ones. As indicated, avoidance and elimination from your environment may be the best solution in many cases.

Reading labels is appropriate, but the New York Poison Control Center estimated that eighty-five percent of product warning labels are inadequate or incorrect. The following are just a few examples of common household products that can be toxic.

❖ **Sodium hypochlorite** - Common laundry bleach! Most people never experience problems with this compound, but if mixed with toilet bowl cleaners or other acidic compounds, it can be very dangerous because poisonous chlorine gas is released. Oxygen-based alternatives are available and are not toxic. The product Borax is also useful as a whitening agent.

- **Naphthalene or paradichlorobenzene** - Used in moth crystals and moth balls, both carcinogenic. Alternatives are garment bags or tight fitting boxes.
- **Methylene chloride** - Used as paint stripper. Carcinogenic when breathed or handled.
- **Toluene** - Used as solvent in many products including paints. Can result in birth defects.
- **Trisodium nitrilotriacetate (NTA)** - Ingredient in some laundry detergents. Carcinogenic.
- **Xylene** - Used in some adhesives, spray paints, and scuff removers. Reproductive and neurotoxin.
- **2-butoxyethanol** - Used as solvent in carpet and other cleaning solutions. Toxic to the liver and kidneys and may cause blood disorders.
- **Perfluorinated chemicals (PFC)** - Used to make non-stick surfaces and stain repellants. Can result in developmental problems in children and may cause cancer.
- **Perchloroethylene (Perc)** - Used in dry cleaning and found in newly dry-cleaned clothing. Neurotoxin may cause dizziness, memory loss, drowsiness, and loss of coordination.
- **Polyvinyl Chloride (PVC)** - Type of plastic used to make such things as pipes, shower curtains, bottles, imitation leather, window blinds, window frames, and flooring. Toxic to liver, lungs, and nervous system. Can cause reproductive problems.

The above list is certainly not complete, but it makes one aware that toxins exist, even in the home. By becoming aware, one can engage in the elimination and avoidance of those substances. By becoming proactive, one is taking another step toward a healthier life for oneself and one's families.

There is another interesting topic that escapes attention simply because it has become an "accepted" part of everyday life. I'm speaking of the addition of fluoride to our water system. The question remains, why is this health menace still an integral part of every community in this country? In 1950, the U.S. Public Health Service endorsed putting fluoride in the water supply to prevent tooth decay. Believe it or not, the recommendation was made without the support of a single trial! Does it actually accomplish what those short-sighted individuals claimed, or is it causing more problems than it has solved? As with many government recommended programs, it is a disaster! Proponents of water fluoridation will not debate this issue in an open forum and continue to rely upon the fact that most people will remain ignorant about this issue. As a science-based doctor, I would NEVER prescribe anything for a patient I had not met and examined. Not only would that be preposterous, but it would simply be practicing bad medicine. That has happened with the fluoridation of water! Every person that drinks water from a public source will consume it the rest of their lives whether they want it or not. In a supposedly free country, how could that have happened? Furthermore, why is it still happening? It **has not been effective** in reducing the incidence of tooth decay as noted by one of the largest studies ever undertaken on this issue.[1] Furthermore, we now know that fluoride is only effective when used topically, not systemically! That means that it does nothing when ingested, such as with drinking fluorinated water, but can be effective when applied to the teeth.[2] As a result, why are we still forced to drink water from a public source that is fluorinated? If anyone wishes to use fluoride topically, as with toothpaste containing fluoride, then that becomes the person's choice and becomes a non-issue for every other person who chooses not to use it topically. It's easy, it's individualized, and it doesn't infringe upon those who choose otherwise! If fluoride was an inert substance that did not have the potential for causing health problems, the fluoridation of water would be more palatable and cause less concern. However, that is not the case! Fluorine is a halogenated atom and belongs to the same chemical class as chlorine, **iodine,** and bromine. When fluoride combines with another element, such as sodium, it forms a compound. In the example, it would then be called sodium fluoride. Since fluorine is in the same class of elements called halogens, the other halogens behave in a similar manner. That is one of the major problems of putting fluoride in the water supply. We are in the midst of a hypothyroid (low thyroid function) epidemic and iodine is essential for the formation of thyroid hormones Since fluorine is in the same class with iodine, one can begin to understand how this element can act as a substitute for iodine in the formation of T3 and T4 hormones. Also consider the fact that another prevalent halogen, chlorine (in a compound form), is put in our water supply for purification. I think it's really commendable that our government spends so much of their time trying to protect us from the ravages of tooth decay and infections, but it's not such a good idea when one considers the many health problems created as a result. Review the chapter on hypothyroidism and determine for yourself whether you would prefer to keep fluoride in the water even though it doesn't work or take it out of the water to prevent thyroid health problems. Actually, it doesn't require a great deal of logic to reach the proper conclusion, but most reading this have fallen for the myths perpetrated by the proponents of water fluoridation. I think this madness should be stopped, but it will take public pressure for that to happen. It's simply amazing to me how so many lies continue to be accepted as the truth.

Consider the following scenario: you visit your doctor at which time you are advised to start drinking a daily mixture composed of ten percent methanol (wood alcohol), fifty percent phenylalanine (neuroexcitatory amino acid), and forty percent aspartic acid (another neuroexcitatory amino acid). Wood alcohol is not the same as ethanol that is found in alcoholic beverages. It has a different chemical formula, but it's the breakdown of methanol that is important. Wood alcohol (methanol) is slowly metabolized and changes into formaldehyde and formic acid.[3] Formaldehyde is used to preserve laboratory tissue specimens and as embalming fluid by morticians. It is highly toxic and is stored in body cells. It can damage DNA, it is highly neurotoxic, and is a known stimulant for the development of cancer cells. Formic acid is the substance that causes the pain from ant bites and it is also a neurotoxin. Some people have a condition known as phenylketonuria (PKU) that results from the inability to metabolize the amino acid, phenylalanine. As a result, they must be very careful not to consume anything containing that substance. For those without PKU, the consumption of neuroexcitatory amino acids is not typically a problem unless that consumption is more than the body requires or if they are consumed without other amino acids. Higher levels of neuroexcitory amino acids have been linked to the development of ADHD and other neurocognitive disorders. If the above noted scenario were to take place, what would your response be? You would think your doctor had gone off the deep end! Why would any sane person recommend the consumption of poisonous and other potentially harmful substances? The point is, you are probably already consuming such a substance, but were unaware. It is called **aspartame** and is marketed under the trade names **Equal®, Nutrasweet®, Spoonful®, Benevia®, and NatraTaste®.** It was initially developed by accident and was submitted to the FDA as an alternative sweetener to sugar. However, we now know that it actually stimulates the appetite and can result in weight gain. It is an ingredient in many foods, beverages, drugs, and toothpastes. All told, it is in over 9,000 products. How is this **silent toxin** allowed to remain available for consumption?

Why did the FDA approve this substance in the first place after not getting approval for over eight years? It came about as the result of politics and payoffs instead of science. Donald Rumsfeld, who was to later become a member of George W. Bush's cabinet (Secretary of Defense), took over as the president of **G.D. Searle** in 1977. It was G.D. Searle that developed aspartame. Even though aspartame had known dangerous effects, Rumsfeld pushed for approval through the

FDA. Arthur Hull Hayes was appointed as commissioner of the FDA during the administration of President Ronald Reagan, and he was able to force approval of aspartame in July 1981 because of his position. It has been alleged that several people were simply paid off as well, including government attorneys who were supposed to be investigating irregularities about aspartame. In 1985, G.D. Searle sold out to chemical giant **Monsanto,** who created the **Nutrasweet Company** as a separate entity.[4]

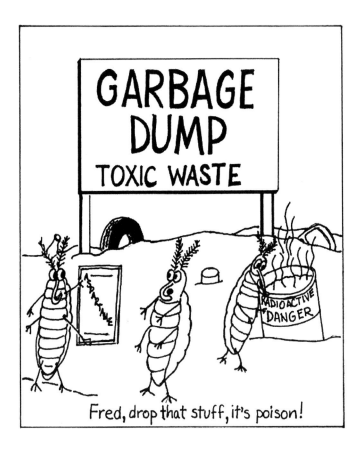

A number of supposedly reputable organizations, including the **AMA (American Medical Association)**, issued statements supporting the use of aspartame. Unbelievable as it sounds, the very organizations that are supposed to be gatekeepers for our health, have caved in and allowed this dangerous substance to remain on our shelves and in our foods and beverages. There is a great deal more dirty-dealing with this story, but suffice it to say that we have a silent toxin in our midst because of dirty politics and payoffs. In order to avoid this dangerous toxic substance, you must read labels and avoid anything containing aspartame.

Our discussion would be incomplete if I omitted toxins contained in many cosmetics and personal products. I obviously don't have the space to list every single cosmetic or personal care product that contains toxins, but a few specifics are in order and will hopefully succeed in making the reader more aware and cautious. I discussed the silent killer, aspartame, and how it metabolizes to form formaldehyde. Please keep in mind that the FDA approved aspartame for use in humans! Formaldehyde is very toxic and can cause irritation of the skin, eyes, and mucous membranes, as well as the more serious issues of brain damage (neurotoxicity), DNA damage, and cancer. Not only is formaldehyde a metabolite of aspartame metabolism, but it is also used as a preservative in some shampoos, liquid hand cleaners, hair conditioners, shower gels, and even in children's bubble bath. It is used because it is an effective preservative, but mostly because it is cheap. Preservatives are used for the purpose of preventing growth of micro-organisms that could be harmful. Yes, it's an effective preservative, but at what cost? It is not required to be listed on labels when it is simply being used as a preservative. It has a great potential for being toxic, but can remain hidden from consumers because of quirks in the law. There are alternatives available that function as preservatives and have no known toxicity to human beings. The following list specifies a few of the chemicals that are known toxins, but are ingredients in either cosmetics or personal care products:

❖ **Phthalates** - Used as softening agent for plastic or in lotions to provide consistency. Present in most plastics such as shower curtains, bottles, storage containers, toys, plastic bags and food wraps, detergents, vehicle interiors, vinyl flooring, and cosmetics, as well as in personal care products such as perfume, nail polish, soaps, deodorants, hair spray, and shampoos. Can result in developmental problems in children, reproductive problems, and hormonal disruption.

❖ **Triclosan** - Antibacterial used in liquid hand soaps, dish detergents, cleaning products, some toothpastes, toys, and bedding. Can result in endocrine and immune dysfunction.

❖ **Sodium Lauryl Sulfate (SLS) or Sodium Laureth Sulfate (SLES)** - Harsh chemicals used in industry as an engine degreaser that is used in virtually every personal cleaning product such as shampoos, hair conditioners, toothpastes, and body cleansers. Can damage the skin, the eyes, and hair and can form nitrosamines that are known carcinogens.

❖ **MEA, DEA and TEA (mono-, di- and triethanolamine)** - Typically found in products that foam such as bubble bath, soaps, body wash, shampoo, and facial cleanser. Can result in allergic reactions, cause eye irritation, and dry the skin and hair. Can be carcinogenic, particularly for the kidneys and liver when reacting with other compounds to form nitrosamines.[5]

❖ **Imidazolidinyl urea and DMDM hydantoin** – Formaldehyde forming preservatives that can result in chest pain, headaches, joint pain, chronic fatigue, allergies, asthma, dizziness, and insomnia. Can impair the immune response and cause cancer. Found in nail polish, antiperspirants, skin, and hair products.

❖ **Methyl, ethyl, propyl, and butyl parabens** - Used to extend shelf life by inhibiting growth of microbes (germs). Very toxic and can cause allergies and skin rashes.

❖ **F & C color pigments (Coal tar dyes)** - Used for the purpose of adding color to cosmetics and personal care products. Typically labeled as FD7C or D4C and followed by a number. Carcinogenic!

❖ **Isopropyl alcohol-solvent and denaturant** - Found in hand lotions, after shave lotions, fragrances, hair color rinses, and many other cosmetics that can result in nausea, vomiting, headaches, dizziness, depression, narcosis, and coma.

❖ **Propylene glycol (PG)** - Approved and touted to be "safe" by the same agency (FDA) that brought you the **silent toxin,** aspartame. Used as a "wetting" solution in many products, including most forms of make-up, hair care products, deodorants, mouthwash, toothpastes, after shave, and lotions. It is the same chemical used in many antifreeze solutions. It is potentially toxic to the kidneys, liver, and brain.

❖ Other toxic chemicals may not typically be in the home, but many are close by and we come in contact with those as a result of exposure by other means. Some of the examples are in the following list.

❖ **Toxic fertilizer** - As odd and unbelievable as this may seem, many fertilizers are the result of recycling hazardous industrial waste. The steel industry accounts for 30% of the waste that is recycled and used as fertilizer. High levels of zinc are present in hazardous waste from the steel industry, and plants do well with higher levels of zinc added to the soil. However, there are also very toxic heavy metals in those hazardous waste products as well.[6] This is the unbelievable part: the label doesn't list the toxins! Twenty-nine fertilizers, all from different companies in twelve different states, were tested by two separate organizations and **they all tested high for levels of lead, mercury, arsenic, uranium, cadmium, beryllium, chromium, and vanadium.** Each of these metals is either a known or suspected carcinogen, causes reproductive or developmental problems, or is harmful to the liver, kidneys, and blood. It is absolute that arsenic and chromium cause cancer, and it is probable that beryllium and lead cause cancer as well. Lead, cadmium, and mercury are known as persistent bioaccumulative toxins (PBTs) because they persist for long periods in the environment and end up in the tissues of animals and humans.[7]

❖ The reader must understand that these fertilizers are not only being used in the agricultural sector, they are also the same fertilizers being used to maintain public and private foliage and grassy areas. **This might include your own front yard!** One should think twice before allowing children or animals to play freely in that pretty green lawn that resulted from fertilization. These substances must be banned from fertilizers, but until proper monitoring is in place, the process of recycling hazardous industrial waste for use in fertilizer **must be stopped.** At this time, it is virtually impossible to determine the amount of toxins in fertilizer used by lawn companies or those purchased and used by people privately. The same holds true for the farming community. As a result, these many dangerous substances end up being absorbed or in our food supply. Regardless, it is resulting in health problems for us all.

❖ **Polychlorinated biphenyls (PCBs)** –
Compounds formerly used in transformers and capacitors. Banned worldwide (banned in U.S. in 1979) because of neurotoxicity, birth defects, carcinogenesis, liver toxicity, and endocrine dysfunction issues. They are very difficult to destroy resulting in contamination of the atmosphere and water sources from landfills. One can be subjected to PCB toxicity by consuming affected food sources such as pork, chicken, fish, and beef, or by breathing contaminated air. One must avoid areas known to have been contaminated by PCBs.

❖ **Polychorinated dibenzodioxins (dioxins)** - By-product of the manufacturing of organochlorides, the incineration of chloride-containing compounds such as PVCs, the bleaching of paper, certain herbicides, and from natural sources such as forest fires and volcanoes. One of the most well known dioxin containing compounds was Agent Orange that was used as a defoliant in Vietnam. It can cause mutations and malformations by interfering with gene transcription, tumors, nervous system disorders, immune dysfunction, and cancer.

The recognized ill effects of smoking are so well known that one would have to have been locked in a closet for the last fifty years not to have that knowledge. Since the hazards of tobacco smoke have been published many times and since most people know the health risks, I will not take up space to repeat what is already well known. There will always be those in denial who feel that those risks don't apply to them and bad things always happen to other people. Of course, there are those who simply have no concern. I have often heard smokers use the example of a relative, friend, etc. who smoked and lived far into old age. If the story was true, smoking did not affect that person the same way it does the majority of the people. The fact is that toxins don't affect everyone the same way. What many smokers don't seem to understand is that smoke continues to be released and breathed by those around them (secondary smoke exposure). This is supposedly a free country and if a person chooses to smoke, they should be allowed to smoke all they want, as long as they're not blowing it in someone else's face that has chosen to not take that risk!

If smoking caused instantaneous death, that would get even the most diehard smoker's attention, but since the ill effects of inhaling various carcinogens contained in cigarette smoke is cumulative, they continue to smoke thinking they will dodge a bullet. The same holds true for many other toxic compounds in that they also have a cumulative effect. The talking heads for the industries that produce toxin laden products typically use the line of reasoning that the levels of toxins in their products are not high enough to cause problems. It takes varying lengths of time for the damage to occur and that depends upon the toxin and the individual. As an example, review the sweet toxin **aspartame** that is found in hundreds of food products! For those who may enjoy drinking embalming fluid, there's no need to read that again. If toxins caused instantaneous death, there would be little to no problem because most sane individuals would avoid them. There would be such a public outcry that any toxin of that nature would have the word **"POISON"** on the label for all to see or it would be removed from the marketplace. However, in the vast majority of cases, it doesn't happen that way, and by being cumulative toxins, they escape attention. It is not the intent of this chapter to create fear and panic; to the contrary, knowledge is power. Knowledge gleaned from this chapter will provide you the power of choice to avoid many of the above noted compounds that are so prevalent in our environment. Most people are so busy with their everyday lives they never understand the implications of continuing exposure to many of these compounds. As a result of not having the necessary fund of knowledge, they remain complacent and silent. Complacency and silence are two of the main ingredients to ensure this situation doesn't change. The only thing that will bring needed change to save lives and prevent misery is public exposure and pressure brought to bear on those in government whose jobs depend on your vote. It is shameful and dishonorable to continue promoting products that are known to be harmful. It is obvious that the promoters have no honor or integrity and will do nothing to prevent these products from reaching the marketplace unless forced to do so.

My hope is that the reader has gained a new perspective about toxins in our environment as a result of reading this chapter. It's common sense to avoid such compounds, but what does one do as an alternative? One must obviously use products that are not toxic and will not result in health issues. Again, providing alternatives to every toxin in the environment would be a gargantuan task, but I will provide some examples of things you can and should do now. First, *start reading labels and eliminate products* from the home that are known toxins. Secondly, *stop purchasing products, regardless of slick advertising, that contain the toxins listed.* Look for alternatives to products containing known toxins. As an example for those who wish to avoid sugar, but now realize the toxic nature of aspartame, there are viable alternatives. All of the alternatives are better, but many have problems of their own. There is *one relatively unknown* non-toxic natural sweetener that actually tastes like sugar, but does not stimulate an insulin response to any great extent. It is known as **erythritol.** It is available in some health food stores or online. **Stevia** is also non-toxic and a natural sweetener, but regardless of claims, it actually doesn't taste like sugar to me. Perhaps it's my taste buds, but stevia just doesn't do it for me. It doesn't mean that one should not use stevia as a sweetener. Every individual's taste is different and there are people who may prefer stevia over erythritol. There is a product available that contains both erythritol and stevia and it is known as Truvia®. Regardless of what one chooses to use as a sweetener, one now knows the truth about aspartame and the many foods and beverages in which it is used, so use it at one's own peril.

I have spoken of iodine more than once because it is such an important essential element for optimal health, regardless of the opinions based on sham studies. Iodine is necessary for proper functioning of the thyroid, but it is necessary for the proper function of other organ systems as well. It also works as a detoxifying agent, and in view of the many toxins in our environment, iodine is an easy and inexpensive way to protect one's self by helping to eliminate those from the body. Iodine is considered a halide and is in the same chemical class as fluorine and chlorine. Since fluoride and chloride are both added to public water, it is difficult to avoid those potentially toxic compounds without filtering the water. Some household filters are very effective in removing toxins and unnecessary halides from the water. Another alternative is bottled water, but many of those are not as pure as claimed, and most are supplied in plastic bottles in which phthalates have been released. Don't store food or liquids in plastic containers and never heat food in a plastic container as phthalates can be released into the contents. Use glass containers!

Open the window of your automobile, particularly if it has been unoccupied while sitting in the sun. The heat generated results in the release of a number of toxins from the interior components that become airborne. The greasy film that accumulates on the inside of the windshield contains a number of those toxins including phthalates and benzene. Open the windows of your home periodically as well to allow airborne toxins to be eliminated from the air. Keep in mind that the air in your home is typically much more toxic than the outside air. Check for leaks in your home or work place periodically. Persistent leaks result in moisture that can lead to toxic mold formation.

Once you know the facts, it becomes somewhat of a scary thought to use fertilizers, pesticides, and herbicides just to have a green lawn and foliage of which to be proud. There are alternatives to common toxic pesticides and herbicides. I would recommend visiting **seedman.com** as a start on the journey of eliminating toxins from your garden and lawn. Common toxic fertilizers can be replaced with organically derived fertilizers that are free of the toxic compounds listed previously. In some cases, the soil in lawns is very acidic and treatment with simple lime solves the problem of slow or no growth. A number of lawn care centers provide a service of testing your lawn soil for its pH (acid or alkaline). Protecting yourself and your family from toxins begins with knowledge, but the rest is up to you.

Notes

[1] Yiamouyiannis, J, "Water Fluoridation and Tooth Decay: Results from the 1986-1987 National Survey of US Schoolchildren." Journal of the International Society of Fluoride Research, April 1990; 23(2):55-67.

[2] "Laboratory and epidemiologic research suggests that fluoride prevents dental caries predominately after eruption of the tooth into the mouth, and its actions primarily are topical for both adults and children." CDC 1999; MMWR, 48:933-940.

[3] Monte, WC, "Aspartame:Methyl alcohol and the public health." J Appl Nutr, 1984;36:42-54.

[4] http://www.aspartamekills.com and www.wnho.net

[5] Cosmetic Ingredient Review, Washington DC, 1996 CIR Compendium

[6] "Factory Farming: Toxic Waste and Fertilizer in the United States, 1990-1995." Environmental Working Group, 1998.

[7] "Visualizing Zero: Eliminating Persistent Pollution in Washington State." Washington Toxics Coalition, 2000.

ABOUT THE AUTHOR

Dr. Ken Knott received his medical education and earned a Doctor of Medicine degree from the University of Tennessee in 1976. He then completed a rotating surgical internship in Phoenix, Arizona through the Good Samaritan Hospital System, and an additional year training at the regional Spinal Cord Injury Center that included a rotation through one of the very first chronic pain treatment centers in the country. It was during his time in Phoenix that Dr. Knott first became aware of prolotherapy, otherwise known as regenerative injection therapy (RIT).

While in Phoenix, Dr. Knott was hired to serve in the capacity of track doctor at Phoenix International Raceway. During his stint, he developed a keen interest in automobile racing that he pursued. After competing as an amateur for six years, he began racing professionally that ultimately resulted in him becoming a regular driver in the highly touted IMSA racing series driving a Grand Touring Prototype race car. Not only did he compete, but he made his way to the winning podium on several occasions. Needless to say, Dr. Knott is not your typical doctor.

After finishing his training in Arizona, Dr. Knott then relocated to Columbus, Ohio in order to train at Ohio State University where he was fortunate enough to be accepted into the prestigious and world-renowned program of Physical Medicine and Rehabilitation (PM&R). Upon completion of his residency training, Dr. Knott remained on staff as a clinical instructor, but also established a private practice. He was awarded board certification in PM&R and continued his practice of diagnosing and treating many neurological and musculoskeletal conditions.

Dr. Knott subsequently moved his medical practice to his present location in Marietta, Georgia in 1988. He became very active in the American Association of Orthopaedic Medicine which he had joined upon its inception in 1983. Dr. Knott served as president from 2000 to 2002 and he continued to serve on the AAOM Board of Directors and chaired the marketing committee through 2009. He has been a speaker on many occasions, not only for the AAOM, but other medical and non-medical groups as well. He was instrumental in the planning and implementation of numerous medical workshops and meetings and served as the annual conference chairman for the AAOM in 2000.

For many years, Dr. Knott personally witnessed how medical myths and incorrect standards of care resulted in avoidable illnesses and misery. As a result, he authored this fact-based book in which he dispels popular medical myths and rumors about living a longer, healthier life. There are a variety of thought-provoking subjects, including those about bioidentical hormone replacement, he has made easy to understand.

www.managingyourage.com